A Survivor's Guide to Breast Cancer

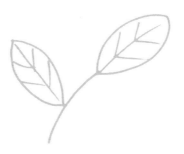

Alice F. Chang, Ph.D.,
with Karen Mang Spruill, M.A.

NEW HARBINGER PUBLICATIONS, INC.

Grateful acknowledgment is made to the following publishers for reprinted material:

Breast form photographs and color/sizing chart and text are reprinted with permission of Colorplast Corporation, Amoena Divison, Marietta, Georgia, 1995-1999

Photographers:

First photograph: Jon Wolf of Jon Wolf Photography Tucson, Arizona (12/1993)

Back Cover Photograph: Norma Rider of Portrait Connections Tucson, Arizona (1999)

Facility Photographs are with permission from Southern Arizona Cancer Center (1999) and Alice Rae's (1999), Tucson, Arizona

Medical records photographs Chuck Heidenreich Tucson, Arizona (1999)

Photo sequence of the body as it underwent treatment taken by friends and family (1994-1999) Jones Photo, Tucson, Arizona

Illustrations 1-4: by Darlene Nawrocki: The Graphic Solution, Chicago, Illinois

Designs for pins: The Graphic Solution, Chicago, Illinois

Publisher's Note

A Survivor's Guide to Breast Cancer describes Alice F. Chang's personal experiences with breast cancer. This book does not provide specific medical and/or psychological advice to breast cancer patients and should in no way be a substitute for appropriate care. This book is intended for use as a supplemental resource by patients and their families before, during, and after the treatment process.

This publication is designed to provide accurate and authoritative information in regard to the subject matter covered. It is sold with the understanding that the publisher is not engaged in rendering psychological, financial, legal, or other professional services. If expert assistance or counseling is needed, the services of a competent professional should be sought.

Contents

Acknowledgments

This volume, and indeed my survival, would not have been possible without the support, advice, insight, and generosity of friends and colleagues far too numerous to mention. To all those who do and those who do not find themselves named in the text, especially my many gracious colleagues across the nation, and the caring staff members at the American Psychological Association, please know you have my deepest gratitude.

I continue to draw inspiration and sustenance from my fellow cancer survivors, from the courageous fallen, and from the friends and families whose lives have been touched by cancer.

I am touched by the courage and generosity of all those who have permitted us to share their stories in these pages and have asked to remain anonymous. Thanks to Angela Wu and to Norma V. Martinez, both of whom had cancer at the same time I did and whose stamina, fortitude, and love within their families and among the young children will forever be an inspiration to me.

The following professionals have provided countless hours of their valuable time and expertise. I offer particularly profound and enduring gratitude to my own "team": My psychologist, who will remain anonymous, U. Venessa Roeder, M.D. (surgeon), Robert J. Brooks, M.D. (oncologist), Edward E. Rogoff, M.D. (radiologist), David S. Goldman, M.D.

(pathologist), Mark Goldstein, male breast cancer survivor who helped with question and answer appendix, and Jay T. Peterson, M.D. (consultant/friend). Without them and their staff members, I would not be here today to share this story.

Finally, I offer special thanks to my friend, Paul Donnelly, who initially inspired me to talk and write about my illness to help others as we collaborated on *Trees Don't Mourn the Autumn*, a play about many aspects of my life including my experience with breast cancer.

Ms. Spruill wishes to offer additional thanks to Dr. Timothy Spruill, the computer tech, and to salute the memory of "Aunt Florence" Baldwin, the first woman she knew with a mastectomy and one who lived life with great love. She also wishes to thank all those women who have urged us to hurry and finish the book because they know someone who needs it.

This book is dedicated to A.N. Reich and to my brother G. W. Chang, his family and the memory of my sister-in-law, Wai Lin Chang.

Introductions

When I began researching this book, I found fifty-two books in print about breast cancer by women who had a close brush with it. There were no books about Asian women with breast cancer. The common myth is that Asians don't get breast cancer. I am living proof that this is not the case. In this book it is my goal to provide all readers with a clear idea of what to expect and how to cope. I also recognize and address the needs of single women, as well as those in relationships. I hope to provide those in similar circumstances with support and information. As a clinical psychologist writing from a personal and professional point of view, I will not be quoting statistics or exploring academic issues. Rather, I will provide practical information to help patients, their families, and professionals cope with cancer.

Many women hear the term "breast cancer" and even have friends who have experienced mastectomy, but few have seen the process. I felt compelled to take many photographs during the entire timeline of diagnosis, treatment, and recovery. At the time I thought it would be good for my memory. Some of these are included in this book, not to shock or scare anyone into health care, but because women need to know what the procedures look like. Even more importantly, people working with and relating to a woman in treatment need to know, in a tangible form, how it looks and feels. Many women never show their bodies to their loved ones again, out of fear of what they might think. In my practice I have seen clients who are healthy survivors of breast cancer who have not shown their bodies to anyone, except reluctantly to their physician, for up to five years after the surgery. I have found in my work with clients, that given information, they have greater choices. This book provides information to facilitate choices for people involved in the healing process.

Breast cancer is a chronic disease. There are coping skills that you can use to get through it. Techniques used to manage other traumatic situations can work with breast cancer also. This is where the breast cancer experience generalizes into other life experiences. Generalizing from specific experiences can provide a foundation applicable to many other experiences.

This is what I do for a living. I work with people who have chronic diseases. I teach them how to adjust to their illnesses, to keep going, to keep a positive attitude, and to look at things realistically.

The golden rule in my office is: *If you can do something about it, let's do it; if you cannot, let's put it aside.* And if it comes up again and you can do something, do it, and if you cannot, put it aside. This is also the golden rule of this book.

Alice F. Chang, Ph.D.

Lumps are scary things. Women are now trained to search and destroy lumps—to take them seriously and view them as the enemy. Lumps can indicate cancer or deformity. So of course, it's difficult to be calm and unruffled about lumps, especially when they hurt. Alice had a painful lump and was told that it couldn't be cancer. I have had fibrocystic breast lumps and more recently benign multiple lipomas (fatty tumors). I was told that lipomas shouldn't hurt, yet mine did, which increased my anxiety.

A few years ago after having a lipoma in my leg excised, I called a female acquaintance whom I knew had survived breast cancer. I wanted to know what she had learned from her illness, and frankly I thought that a cancer survivor might be the only person with whom I could relate because of my new lumpiness. My friend and I had lunch together. She gave me courage as she explained how she had vowed to take her health into her own hands. We talked about doctors and second opinions, diet and supplements. It seemed so comforting to talk with another woman who knew firsthand about having a body that went berserk and betrayed her. After we talked, I also knew that someday I wanted to share the courage that she had given me with other women.

I have always been fascinated with people's stories of conquering illness. Some women retreat into a kind of denial after having cancer or a severe illness. They don't want to relive the trauma—they just want to go on with life. Perhaps they fear that if they talk about their experience they will be perceived as whiners. But we know from research that talking and writing about traumatic events can relieve stress and help us grow. There is a context for every illness and we need to talk about what an illness means to us. Doctors would do well to pay attention to what a condition means to the woman, not just what the textbook describes for that condition.

Since the lipomas I hadn't even attempted regular breast self-exams. I mentioned my concern about recurring lipomas to my former physician and during an exam she said, "You sure do have lumpy breasts." I figured that I wouldn't be able to tell a malignant lump from the others. Recently, I changed physicians and my new doctor talked to me about the hard, gritty nature of a "bad lump" compared to the round or soft nature of lipomas. She wasn't going to let me off the hook so easily. And she even acknowledged that, indeed, lipomas could hurt. She was the first doctor to tell me that.

Alice's story and her vulnerability have also changed my life, and I am privileged to help share her story. Now I'm more dedicated to my regular mammograms, attempting self-exams, and talking to my teenage daughter about breast lumps. We want to assist other people in discovering healing and health. There is strength in telling our stories.

Karen Mang Spruill, M.A.

Chapter One

Faulty Assumptions

We all make assumptions. They can be based on everything from cultural values to advice from friends. Assumptions can hinder communication and slow down response time to certain problems or events. Before being diagnosed with breast cancer, I held some faulty assumptions about its symptoms.

Return to Tucson

September 1992—Kansas City in the rearview mirror. After seventeen years in the Midwest, I was looking forward to returning to Tucson as a form of semiretirement. Having recently had a bout with chemical sensitivities, which left me gasping for air, I desperately needed a fresh start. Early in my career as a psychologist, I had been an assistant professor at the University of Arizona. While there, I had helped to establish a health clinic for Native Americans. I had also worked on parent-training programs and treatment programs for recovering alcoholics. After leaving my teaching position, I set up a private practice in Kansas City. At first I worked mostly with those suffering from eating disorders and alcoholism. Soon I began taking on clients who were coping with a variety of chronic physical ailments, including orthopedic problems, renal dysfunction, seizure disorders, and cancer. By 1979, people suffering from some type of chronic illness comprised 90 percent of my client base.

In the ensuing years I had reached many of the demanding professional goals that I had set for myself. I had been a professor of psychology, staff psychologist at medical facilities, director of a pain clinic, an active member of both local and national psychological associations, and I had run a bustling private practice. I was looking forward to a lower profile and a slower pace, as a visiting scholar in the Department of Psychology at the University of Arizona. Working with a friend and colleague, I would begin a series of research projects.

My little Italian greyhound, Vivi, and I would be braving it alone, as we had become used to doing. Vivi was born in 1988. I rescued her from an abusive environment and we were buddies in and out of the consultation room. My clients (for the most part) loved her. We were certainly going to miss the good friends we had made in Kansas City, but it was time to move on.

With little financial cushion, I had to carefully consider all the expenses of my new life. In 1989, I had found a comfortable home in a pleasant, affordable neighborhood. After several months of shopping for health insurance, I had resolved to invest in the best plan that I could find. I reminded myself that if I ever became seriously ill I would not get a second chance. Like everyone, I had to carefully weigh how much my being well was worth. After all, I was self-sufficient and the bills and the buck stopped with me.

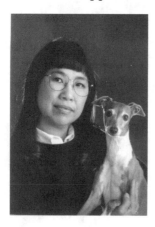

Me and Vivi

The months passed quickly as I reacquainted myself with the campus and community. I elected to work with substance abuse and domestic violence issues among Southeast Asian refugee families. I wanted to do some service work and learn if I could influence policy and law for treatment with these new community members.

A Painful Lump

During the summer of 1993 I began an exercise program to tone my muscles and strengthen my respiratory system, which had been damaged by chemical sensitivities. I was soon to begin a three-year tenure on the American Psychological Association's Board of Directors, and was currently serving on several committees and task forces. Proud of my resolve, I maintained my workouts in a hotel during an APA meeting in Washington, D.C. Sometime in November I noticed pain in the back and rib muscle area on my left side. I assumed that I had strained some muscles while exercising at the hotel. Despite my commitment, I thought it best to lay off the workout regimen. In December I realized that the pain was still there. Also, my normally smaller left breast was suddenly larger than my right one. I noticed a lump a little smaller than a golf ball that was causing my breast to sag a bit.

I talked and even joked with some women friends and colleagues about it: "Hey, I'm fifty years old and my breast is growing!" Some laughed and said, "You must have terrible fibroids." A family member explained that at my age many women develop fibroid cysts associated with menopause. Someone also mentioned that it was a good sign that I had pain, since there was no pain with breast cancer. I kept scanning my memory for how my former cancer clients had experienced their initial symptoms. I was relieved that I could not remember anyone who had pain with their lumps.

A friend once told me about his sixty-four-year-old colleague and the man's fifty-eight-year-old wife. The couple had noticed "something" about the wife's breast but figured that it was "the change." They continued to ignore a rapidly growing tumor until it began breaking through the tissue and skin, causing bleeding on the surface. I told my friend that this sounded very serious to me and that it was important that they seek medical attention immediately. My friend soon reported that he had talked with them and that they had promised to make a doctor's appointment, although they still did not think it was anything to worry about. I cried inside. I knew that there was something seriously wrong, and that it was already late in the process. The couple did go to see her primary-care physician. After examining her, the physician told the woman that she had cancer even before referring her for a mammogram. They had to wait weeks to complete tests and begin treatment. During this time the couple became frantic. They needed someone to walk them through the steps of this process, even if they could not absorb all that they would be told. I received a dinner invitation to discuss my case with them, since I had already gone through that part of treatment. Getting the right information from a credible person as soon as possible is crucial. Like me, this couple had made some assumptions that proved wrong. Luckily, I did not wait as long to question my assumptions.

Time for a Mammogram

In early December 1993, I made an appointment with a gynecologist and then set out to find the best place in Tucson for a mammogram. I asked everyone I knew, "What is the best mammography place in town?" Nearly everyone replied, "The Cerelle Women's Center." So I did some homework and made an appointment with them. The Cerelle Center had a reputation as the top diagnostic center for breast cancer in the United States. I was scheduled to see a gynecologist on December 29 and the mammogram was scheduled for the following day. I recalled my last mammogram at around age forty-five. I reviewed the results. Sure enough, the screening was normal. But now my left breast was definitely getting bigger, and the pain was getting worse. Also, I recalled the self-exams I conducted. Like many women, I am very body-shy. In my traditional Asian-American family I was taught that the body was for productive function, and not to be touched or seen. Not surprisingly, my self-exams were rather cursory.

When it came time for my gynecology appointment, I was still having a pretty heavy menstrual flow. So, I called to postpone it. When I asked if I should go ahead with the mammogram without seeing the doctor first, the office nurse told me to proceed. I rescheduled the gynecology appointment for late January 1994.

On December 30 I arrived at the Cerelle Center for my mammogram. They had reminded me to not apply deodorant or lotion because it would interfere with the X-ray image. The center was nicely decorated and they even provided colorful gowns instead of the standard paper ones. The atmosphere was light and open with lots of reading material on health and nutrition. Clearly they had paid

When I asked clients if they conducted self-exams or if they knew how, in recent years the answer was usually "Yes." When it was not, I sent them to be trained by the nursing staff of their gynecologist. Some of my clients, though, found it distasteful to "feel" themselves, unless there was a history of breast cancer in the family, and even then it could make for some difficult conversation. The women of strict religious upbringing, who had been taught not to touch their intimate body parts, carried tremendous guilt. In some cases, it caused very late diagnosis of the cancer. For those who had trouble with self-exam, I often suggested that they repeat some phrases designed to help them to think differently about this procedure. For example, "I want to be sure my body is healthy," "As long as I am still here, I need to take care of myself," and "I want to take care of myself" were usually good starting points. Because thoughts generate feelings, we would start by changing their thoughts.

close attention to detail. This thoughtfully decorated room had a comforting effect on me. After giving my medical history, I changed out of my clothes and put on a gown. As I waited for the technician, I noticed a fluffy white stuffed animal on the

Breast self-exam is a must. Like many women, I was originally taught to explore the breast in a concentric circular pattern. More recently, I learned of the MammaCare system. The training for this technique begins with a model breast being constructed specifically for the individual. This serves as a useful comparative tool for examining any future changes in the breast. The examination is then performed in a vertical strip fashion that allows very small abnormalities to be detected.

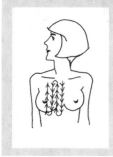
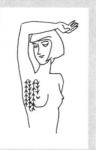

X-ray platform. I learned that it held an internal heating pad and thermostat to keep the platform at about body temperature.

Mammograms come in two basic varieties: those for regular screening and those for diagnostic evaluation, such as mine. The technician told me that she would not take unnecessary pictures but would take as many as needed. The X-ray apparatus was in good working order so that there was no slipping of the guides and the procedure was relatively painless—as painless as you can feel with your breast smashed between two pieces of plastic, horizontally and then vertically! My left breast felt heavier to the technician also. She had some difficulty because it was too dense to photograph; nothing showed up on the image. Eventually she took a couple of pictures with a balloon on the breast to help flatten it and magnify the image so it was less dense. The normally twenty-minute procedure took about an hour. Both the technician and I were assured that the best possible pictures had been taken. She took four photos on the right side and ten on the left.

With nothing officially "wrong" with me, I left for Phoenix in early January on a business trip. I stayed very busy for the next several days. Although the pain in my breast had not subsided, I didn't give the mammogram much thought. I even enjoyed a two-night visit with friends.

A Visit with the Gynecologist

I returned to Tucson late on a Wednesday afternoon. I picked up my mail and unpacked before checking my phone messages. To my surprise and alarm two calls were from the gynecologist's office:

Monday morning: "Hi, Dr. Chang, this is Dr. Jones' office. Wouldn't you like to come in a little early? We want to see you before January 30."

Tuesday afternoon: "Hello, Dr. Chang. Where are you? The doctor would like to see you . . ." I made a mental note to call the doctor's office when I got to work on Thursday morning.

Thursday morning there was yet another message from them at my office. "Gee," I thought to myself, "something must really be wrong." Afraid to call, I busied myself with work. When I finally summoned the courage to pick up the phone, I was given an appointment for the following Monday, January 11. I worked all weekend. I was worried, yet convinced that I just had a fibroid that needed to be aspirated.

With telephone interviews and grant applications to complete, it was not easy for me to squeeze in a doctor's appointment. Still, I arrived at Dr. Jones' office a few minutes early to fill out paperwork. I was then ushered into an exam room where I changed into a gown. File in hand, a doctor who appeared to be in his mid-forties introduced himself and then abruptly asked, "Who are you?"

"I'm Alice Chang."

"I don't know you—why haven't I seen you before?" He was obviously yet inexplicably upset about getting my mammogram.

"I know you don't know me," I retorted. "I had an appointment to see you the day before the mammogram, but my period started and your nurse told me to reschedule my exam and go ahead with the mammogram."

I realized that this was just like many of my clients' complaints that their physician did not listen to his or her staff, or the staff was too busy to keep the physician informed. I told myself not to feel discouraged and to be patient—I had not done anything wrong. In their distress, patients often blame themselves when their dealings with physicians don't go smoothly.

The doctor acknowledged that the Cerelle Center was a good place, and then commented that I would not remember anything that he said (repeating this several more times to my irritation). "I don't make any bones about this," he said. Then he thrust a piece of paper into my hand. "The report says: 'mammogram of the right breast reveals no specific abnormalities. But the left breast . . .'—see that word that is underlined . . . it says 'malignant.'"

Malignant was the only word I saw. The report also said, "We did not inform the patient of the mammographic findings." So of course, I did not know the results before he saw me.

Then he explained mammograms to me, and the odds of a false positive. He reminded me that it was only one diagnostic measure—"You'll need a biopsy to reach a conclusive diagnosis. I know a good surgeon that I'll call for you after the pap exam." He called the nurse into the room, completed the pap culture, and did a quick breast exam (not as thorough as I had experienced with other physicians). He then told me to get dressed while he called to make arrangements with the surgeon. I knew he was not happy with me, though I wasn't sure why. I tried to overlook his attitude because I had heard that he had recently had a family crisis.

I dressed and waited for a long time, until I finally stepped into the hallway. Because his office door was slightly ajar, I could hear him talking on the phone. The surgeon was out of town. Clearly frustrated, he instructed the nurse to give me another surgeon's name so I could make an appointment. I forked over ninety dollars for our five minutes together and left.

I knew that lots of my cancer patients saw insensitive doctors all the time. One of the things I always tell my clients is, "If you feel uncomfortable talking to your doctor and you can't talk to him or her straight, change your doctor." I left knowing I would not see him again. I also suspected that I would not like the surgeon he was referring me to.

A few tips for assembling your medical team:

1. Ask friends and colleagues for names of doctors.
2. Check out the reputation and training for every doctor on your team.
3. Call doctors' offices and ask questions about their credentials and experience.
4. Find the person who is best in his or her field and find out what his or her personality is like.
5. Psychologists and counselors can help take care of your emotional needs. When looking for a therapist, find out how much expertise he or she has with health issues and breast cancer.

The Search for a Surgeon

So I did what I now tell my clients to do. I called everyone I knew who had any connection with a breast cancer survivor in Tucson, and asked them to recommend a good breast surgeon. Within twenty-four hours I had narrowed the selection down to two surgeons. Top on the list was Dr. Yoder. To the gynecologist's credit, that was the surgeon that he had tried, unsuccessfully, to refer me to. I sensed that the need for a surgeon might be urgent, so I picked the next doctor who was a woman and came highly recommended by her patients. I wanted my surgeon to be a woman because I knew I would feel less intimidated by her. Like some other female patients, I was concerned that I could not be as assertive as I needed to be with a male doctor. I also suspected that a woman would be more sensitive to some of the issues confronting me. Dr. Vanessa Roeder, the second best breast cancer surgeon in town, was now the best breast cancer surgeon in town. I also asked the Cerelle Center to fax me a copy of my report so that I could start to absorb the information in it.

I had done enough research on handling the initial diagnosis of a tumor to know that I was missing one essential element. Information is the single most important factor in diminishing psychological trauma for patients. Information was currently in short supply. On Monday night I was restless and uneasy and my dreams were filled with images of my former clients. I dreamed about a client who had a double mastectomy. I saw her laying in her hospital bed. Her body was withering away but her perfectly reconstructed breasts remained. She told me, "I'm going now." I responded by encouraging her to tell her husband and daughter how much she loved them. "Have a nice journey," was the last thing I said to her. I also dreamed that I was running down a long, dark hallway. I could see rows and rows of beds with people who smelled bad and were waiting to die. Terrified and disoriented, I awoke in a sweat. It was not difficult to figure out where some of these images came from. In the late seventies I had worked on the experimental cancer drug unit at a VA hospital. Prior to that, I had worked on a study concerning the chronic mentally ill. In the morning I remembered the more positive patients I had seen over the last fifteen years. Some of them were still alive. I thought about the surgeons and the oncologists who trusted me to work with their patients and their patients' families. I thought about all the conflict that cancer causes families because of the uncertainties and the ambivalent feelings that surround it.

Thankfully, that afternoon I had an appointment with my psychologist. We could talk about the medical team selection and my feelings. When I moved to Tucson in 1992 I had made a serious commitment to therapy. I had worked very hard on some difficult personal issues and we had developed a solid therapeutic alliance.

I had already shared a little of my anxiety about my breast growing and hurting with my psychologist. He strongly encouraged me to get it checked even when I was afraid that my newly acquired insurance would not cover it. Even though I trusted him, I still feared that I could say the wrong thing and cause him to reject me. We discussed the medical team. I shared not only my fears, but my strong urge to deny what was happening. I talked about my need to get grant proposals finished because I needed money to make house payments. At the same time, I added, it would be a good time to die. After all, I had no responsibilities to clients, no immediate family obligations, and my dog would have a good home with friends. I am not sure what all I shared in that hour. One thing I remember clearly, though, was my psychologist saying, "Alice, it's okay with me if you want to bury yourself in your work to cope with the emotional reaction, but don't let this get in the way of proper treatment." He was gently urging me to make the appointment with Dr. Roeder. "And," he added, "when you call, tell them you are *Dr.* Chang." I'm sure I paled. I never told anyone I was a "doctor," as I felt that it was unfair to pull rank. He assured me that I would get treated with more respect. I left saying that I would think about it. That was *all* that I thought about for the next few hours.

By noon I had called the insurance company to find out if Dr. Roeder was on their provider list. I breathed a sigh of relief when I learned that she was. I dialed her number immediately. The nurse patiently answered each of my many questions. She suggested an appointment on February 7. "Okay," I said, but then reminded myself that this might be more urgent. I mentioned that I had acquired a copy of my mammogram report. I read the report over the phone and asked an important question: "Does it make any difference if I have a mammogram that says *malignant tumor*?"

"If the doctor should have an opening in the next day or two do you think you could make it in?" she responded.

"Yeah, I think so."

I left my office phone number. Again, I was reminded that this might be more urgent than I had suspected or wanted to know. By this time, I was really scared. Soon my worst fears might be confirmed.

Being a first-generation Asian-American daughter, the value of hard work in the face of adversity was deeply instilled in me. With a presentation scheduled in a few days, I had plenty to do. That weekend I would leave for the APA's Division Leadership Conference, where I would give a talk on ethnic minorities in governing positions.

That afternoon Dr. Roeder's nurse Jean called to tell me that the doctor had had a cancellation and could see me at four that day. "Since it's such short notice," she asked, "can you pick up the X-rays from the Cerelle Center and bring them

The value of a good insurance plan cannot be exaggerated. After I had met my $500 deductible and started filing claims, my insurance company did a thorough investigation of my medical history. They reviewed all of my records from the past seventeen years. They also got my first mammography report from 1989 that showed a normal result. They ended up paying $100,000 of my $110,000 care. Had I not purchased the very best policy I could afford, I would not have gotten the kind of quality care that I have received. I was charged eighty dollars for my mammogram. When I got my insurance papers, they revealed that the gynecologist had charged me ninety dollars when insurance only allowed him to charge sixty-nine dollars. Two months later I asked his office to return my twenty-one dollars. They conceded that they were in error and immediately sent me a check. Like many patients, I became acutely aware of fees charged the patient versus fees permitted by insurance companies.

along?" Later I realized that the doctor probably didn't have a cancellation but was kind enough to see me at the end of her appointments. Of course that phone call made me anxious, so I continued plugging away at my work. I called my therapist to tell him about the appointment. I knew that he would be as pleased as I would have been for one of my clients.

Late afternoon finally rolled around. I retrieved my records and paid for my mammogram at the Cerelle Center. My insurance was in effect and it had a $500 deductible.

Chapter Two

Betrayed by My Body

I had heard cancer stories from my clients for years. Still, it was a shock to be confronted with it personally. How could this happen to me? I was suddenly thrust into a world of specialists, complicated medical treatments, and critical decisions that I would have to make on my own.

Little Bursts of Light

We stood in the hallway at the surgeon's office, looking at X-rays of my breasts on a lighted background. The growth, which Dr. Roeder called a "tumor" and I called "it," was obvious. She pointed out that the light areas in the X-rays indicated some kind of abnormality. "See these little bursts of light . . . ?"

I recognized the marks and answered, "They're star asterisk clusters."

Dr. Roeder then asked if I knew what they usually indicated, and like a good student I replied, "Sites of calcification."

"That's right. Unfortunately, we don't get asterisks with benign tumors. They are 90 percent true positive for a malignancy. Star asterisks almost always indicate a malignancy."

I enjoyed talking with Dr. Roeder even though I did not like what she had to say. From the moment that she entered

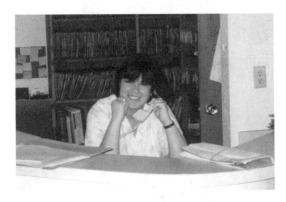

Dr. Roeder's nurse, Jean

the examining room, I liked her confident body language, honest manner, sense of humor, and strong hands. She anticipated a lot of my resistant first-diagnosis responses and even warned me about her cold hands. She knew all the right questions to ask: "What's been going on in your life?" "Is there any history of breast cancer in your family?" "Any trauma to your breast?" "When did this start?" She even demonstrated how each breast had been positioned for the mammogram photographs by squeezing her own breast under her white coat.

While the picture of my right breast contained regular markings and looked normal, the left one was obviously different. Dr. Roeder explained that the tumor was probably toward the central plane of the breast. This is where we both could feel the lump. The angles revealed in the X-rays were fascinating.

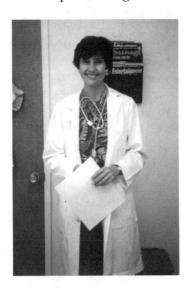

Dr. Vanessa Roeder

The pictures taken with the balloon were clearer yet more diffuse.

With a jolt, I remembered that I was looking at pictures of my own body, not a patient. *I* had arrived earlier, filled out the paperwork, and stood before the nurse as she took a photograph of *me* for the records. I had then undressed my upper body and put on the open-front, plastic-coated paper gown. Dr. Roeder had looked at me and at my naked breasts. She conducted a routine breast exam, except that she seemed to press for every nodule, and explore every inch of the surface. As she was looking at and feeling the left breast lump, she pulled out a ruler and measured it. When I asked her why, she said she liked to check herself against the X-rays, which she hadn't examined yet. Clearly concerned, she told me to go ahead and get dressed, while she looked at the X-rays. Then we looked at them together.

Now Dr. Roeder sat on the examining table while I sat in a chair (reverse from the usual doctor-patient arrangement). "I have never found an easy way to tell a woman that she has cancer. We'll need to confirm with a biopsy, but the indications are very clear. I'm so sorry."

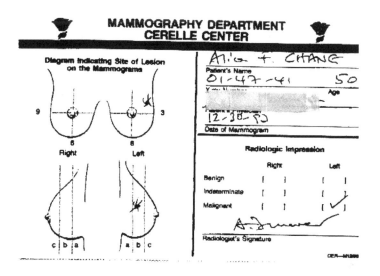

Left and right mammogram

Most cancer patients see their mammograms but do not really look at them since they are in shock or denial. I did not look at mine very well either, but I went back and reviewed them in detail later. In studying the mammogram, the doctors became pretty sure the lymph nodes were involved. As I look back, I had l'orange—orange peel skin. But of course, I had never noticed anything. One of the things about a lot of us women, and me in particular is, we do not look at our bodies. We do not look at our breasts. How would I know I had ripply, rough skin? I'm single. I don't have anyone that looks at my breasts.

Questions and concerns about my career spilled out of me: "I returned to Tucson to increase my research and now I finally have several grant applications in process. I can't get sick now. I just started my practice here. I need to make money so I can pay my deductible . . . and my mortgage! This cannot be happening to me. What am I going to tell people?" Dr. Roeder acknowledged my feelings and fears, and said that she understood my feelings. I believed that she did. She told me about the options for diagnosis and treatment.

"Are you sure it is not a 'fibrous mass,' a cyst or a fibroid? Maybe the mammogram is wrong. The technician took so many pictures—maybe she was new."

"This is an awful shock for you," she said. "But we need to start with a biopsy to remove a tissue sample for microscopic evaluation. There are two kinds of biopsies. The fine-needle biopsy can be done in this office. Like the name suggests, I'll insert a thin needle into the breast and extract some tissue. If we discover that we need a larger sample, then I'll perform an excisional biopsy. As an outpatient, you would probably have that done under a local anesthesia while I would make an incision and remove a bigger tumor sample." She also talked about chemotherapy and radiation. Then she reassured me about preauthorizing any surgery with my insurance.

I told Dr. Roeder that I was leaving on Friday and would not be available until next week. She made a radiology appointment for me with a Dr. Rogoff for Thursday, the day before I would leave for another APA conference. She told me that Dr. Rogoff was friendly and appreciated psychology. She thought that I would like him. She also said that her office would let me know about my appointment with yet another doctor. Dr. Brooks was the oncologist she was referring me to. Because it was already half past five she would have to wait until tomorrow to get in touch with him.

When I arrived home that night there was a message from my psychologist. I was irritated that I had spent so much time with Dr. Roeder that I had missed his call. This compounded the anxiety that I was feeling from my visit with the surgeon. I looked at my big breast and hated it for causing me all of this trouble. I did not know who to talk to, so I did not talk to anyone. Alone and frustrated, I decided that I did not have cancer.

Good Friends, Good Timing

I had only been home a few minutes when the phone rang. It was my friends from Missouri, Robert and Dee Henion. They had an uncanny way of contacting me at critical times in my life. Dee was on the phone and said: "Hi, Alice. Just called to see how you are and let you know our plans . . . what's wrong?" I had met the Henions at an art fair in Kansas City. Robert was a jewelry maker and Dee an artist. They were coming to visit for the International Gem and Mineral Show as they had the previous year. We had had so much fun then. I hated to say anything negative, as I was looking forward to seeing them again. But my voice betrayed me.

"I have a lump in my breast, Dee. I saw a surgeon today and she wants me to get a biopsy—to see if it's cancer. I really like her and she explained everything really carefully."

I began to sing Dr. Roeder's praises. I told her about how straightforward she was and how quickly she set me up with the other doctors. If they were all as bright and competent as she, I was confident I would be well cared for.

We discussed the unrealistic possibility that it wasn't cancer and that the tests would reveal nothing more than a benign growth. After talking with Dee, I felt sad but my anxiety lifted a little. We planned not only to attend the gem and mineral show together, but to celebrate Chinese New Year on February 10, and my birthday a few days later. Through our sadness, we hoped for a positive outcome. They promised to call me in the next week. Talking with Dee had given me courage.

I e-mailed a colleague to cancel an appointment with him. I would have to free up some time for doctor visits. I told him that I had a growth that might be cancer, and had to rearrange my plans. He called and said that his sister had caused him all kinds of anxiety when she had a similar health problem, and it turned out to be nothing. Even though his sister vowed to take better care of herself, she soon lost her resolve. He made it clear that she had wasted his time. I decided not to bother him again.

Sometime on Wednesday I got a call to confirm an appointment with Dr. Brooks, the oncologist, for the following day. Later when my therapist called, I learned that he knew and liked Dr. Rogoff. He assured me that he cared about me and would be there for me (whatever that meant). I was glad to hear from him and that he was concerned. I had done the same for my clients over the years.

On Wednesday morning I called my Kansas City physician's office and asked for his fax number. He is an oncologist, hematologist, and internist who had been my friend and personal physician. He had also sent many patient referrals my way over the years. I had sent him the mammogram report and asked him for an opinion. He called late Wednesday night and explained everything in detail, including what to expect from the radiologist and oncologist. "Alice, this looks like a serious cancer," he added. I did not want to hear that, but listened anyway.

He updated me about various changes in treatments that had occurred over the last few years. We talked a lot and since he was a member of my church in Kansas, he said that they would pray for me.

Meet Dr. . . .

By eleven Thursday morning I was filling out papers in Dr. Rogoff's office. He was a balding man with long, gray hair. His kindness was apparent. He did the "look, feel, see" examination one more time. I wished that I could just hand off the left breast to him. I complained that there was no dignity left, that I was just another pound of flesh. He reminded me that every part of my body was part of me and needed care. He urged me to always feel proud of my body and reminded me that illness does not make the breast bad or alien. "Your body is not the enemy," he insisted. He was very gentle during the examination. His response was surprisingly similar to what mine often was to my clients who so badly wanted to divorce themselves from their bodies. I had never forgotten to remind them of those very words. After I got dressed, we talked. Dr. Rogoff now heard the same kind of rambling that Dr. Roeder did earlier. He was very friendly and I told him about cultural differences and how I did not feel very important in the whole scheme of things. Traditional Asian culture taught "resignation," that women were not important in the big picture. Then I talked about my work with domestic violence in Asian families, and why it was so necessary. I discussed the specifics of my schedule and he seemed confident that everything could work in a timely manner.

We were working on a treatment schedule for chemotherapy, surgery, and radiation and I was still not convinced that I had a tumor, much less cancer! We talked a lot about treatment but it seemed as though we were discussing one of my patients, not me. It was like we were making appropriate plans

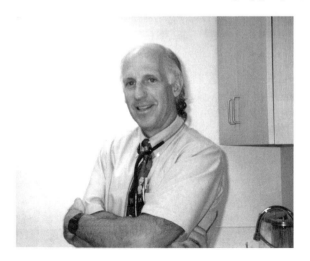

Dr. Rogoff

for another person whom I would be responsible for supporting and caring for.

We also talked about the importance of psychology in the Health Care Reform Act. He was clearly aware of how important psychology is in medical treatment. He had to learn all of his behavioral interventions after his radiology residency, since it was not taught to him in medical school. I reminded him to share his views with his congressional representative and his colleagues.

He introduced me to a social worker who counseled patients and facilitated support groups. We discussed my insurance coverage and my employment status. Dr. Rogoff told me that he would probably see me sometime after I had surgery in June or July (factoring in my travel schedule with surgery around June 21).

Since my home is only three miles from the Cancer Care Center at Tucson Medical Center where I was being treated, I went home for a snack. I talked to Vivi, who had waited in the car while I was in the physician's office. As she eyed my food, I told her about Dr. Rogoff: "I like this radiology guy. Dr. Roeder and my psychologist were right. He seems like an honest, sincerely interested person." He did not act like a know-it-all, as was the case with many radiologists that I had met over the years. So, I had two great people on board so far. Later that day, I was back at the Cancer Care Center filling out papers for Dr. Brooks, the

Since the failure of President Clinton's Health Security Act of 1993, the primary focus of health care reform has been to curb the most egregious abuses of managed care. The need for preventive care, access to care and coverage, portability of coverage, confidentiality, patients' rights, physician autonomy, and the elimination of the "gag" clauses were among the most prominent concerns. The Women's Health and Cancer Rights Act of 1998 offered protection from "drive-through" mastectomies and became law in October of 1998. Mental health professionals continue to advocate for parity for mental health care, support for outpatient mental health care, and protections for the integrity of clinical judgment and standards.

oncologist. The five-oncologist office seemed much less personable than other offices, with many busy, staff members flitting by. I filled out forms and began reading a book on chemotherapy. I was about half done with it by the time I was called in to undress and have my "vitals" taken for the second time that day. Dr. Brooks came in and we talked. He was a large, strong man with a full head of slightly graying hair. I learned that Dr. Brooks was doing some lobbying for the Health Care Reform Act on behalf of some of his fellow oncologists. We discussed both of our busy schedules. Of course, we also talked about chemotherapy and cancer. After examining me, he said that he and Dr. Rogoff agreed that I had "inflammatory carcinoma." The advised course of treatment was "about six chemotherapy treatments, surgery, and radiation." We began to hammer out the treatment schedule. I respected his knowledge and liked his demeanor. He commented that I was reading one of the best books on cancer and even gave me a few others. They would make for important airplane reading the next day when I left for a trip to Washington, D.C. After leaving the exam room, I was ushered into the business office where they asked for payment. I was gripped with shame and embarrassment as I explained that I did not have any money to give them. I had spent my last bit of money at the gynecologist's office on Monday. I gave the office person my insurance card and said that I would have to make payments when I had money.

Another office appointment was scheduled for a week later. Then, he scheduled me for a bone scan, chest X-ray, and blood work. The bone scan was scheduled the following Tuesday, January 18, after my return from Washington, D.C.

The blood work was done in the laboratory next door to Dr. Brooks' offices. I went into a little room furnished with a chair that had a folding armrest, and a small lab table. Barely acknowledging me, the lab tech did a good "stick" on the first try and quickly filled three vials with my blood. I left with a cotton ball on my arm and went to the first floor for my X-ray. Little did I know that I would be visiting this tiny room for years to come, that I would become friendly with the people working in it and used to being stuck for blood samples.

The X-ray waiting room was a very cozy place where three or four patients could be processed at one time. On the day I was there, a temporary employee was struggling to learn how to use the computer. It took her about thirty minutes to get a number for my record. After inputting some additional data, she pushed a key and the screen froze. After about an hour, I suggested that she finish the record the old-fashioned way. She wrote down the remaining information to be entered into the computer later, and I was led into the X-ray room. I had a standard two-view (front and side) chest X-ray and went back to my office.

APA Bound

I needed to get ready for my trip. I had forgotten that I was going to a basketball game between the U of A and Cal-Berkeley. In the early seventies I had been on the faculty of the former school. The game would be a good diversion for me and even though the U of A lost, I had fun. After stopping at my office the next day, I was off to Washington D.C. Once there, I met my former boss from Kansas City and her fiancé for dinner at one of my favorite restaurants. I told her that I might have cancer and was scheduled for a bone scan on Tuesday. As always, I enjoyed her company. It was another good diversion.

The next day was jam-packed with meetings that mercifully saved me from having to discuss my life with anyone. When a couple of people noticed that something was wrong, I told them what was happening and asked them not to talk about it until I knew more. I still clung to the belief that I did not really have cancer. I did not even want to say the word, much less talk about it openly with people. For the rest of the weekend, I told anyone who asked that I felt great and was looking forward to being an official board member in a few weeks. Divulging information was not necessary because "I do not have any data . . . I need to have the bone scan and then I'll have a needle biopsy and I'll be fine."

On Sunday morning shortly before I was to deliver my presentation, I discovered that I had left it on my desk in Arizona, so I had to reconstruct it from memory. My busy subconscious had too much to process! Fortunately, I had sent a large handout to APA Central Office, which had been reprinted, for all the division leaders. Worn out, I returned home on Sunday night and spent the next morning at my office catching up on paperwork and returning calls. My colleague and I were scheduled to have a conference call with a new consultant for my grant proposal. I was anxious about the bone scan.

A Sudden Change in Plans

The phone rang and it was Jean from Dr. Roeder's office. "I just wanted to let you know that you've been scheduled for outpatient surgery at the Ambulatory Surgery Center Tucson Medical Center on Wednesday, seven-fifteen check-in time, and surgery at nine."

I was horrified. I was going to have a slice biopsy, not a needle biopsy. What had gone wrong?

"Does my insurance company approve this kind of procedure?" "Why am I going into the Ambulatory Surgery Center when Dr. Roeder said that she would do the procedure in her office?" "Does this mean that I am going to be anesthetized?" I fired off questions at Jean as fast as they came to me.

Jean said that all the calls had been made and everything had been authorized. I would get gas and to go to "la-la land" for a while. Everything would be fine. Somehow I interpreted this to mean that I would be allowed to watch the surgery, but it would not hurt. I was thinking about laughing gas. I was scared and confused. Dr. Roeder got on the phone and I asked her the same questions: "You told me I was going to have a needle biopsy and you could do it in your office." In fact, she had told me that was *one* of the options. But she had spoken with Dr. Rogoff and Dr. Brooks on Friday, as she said she would, and Dr. Brooks said that he needed a larger specimen to send for hormone receptor and DNA studies. The needle biopsy would not produce a big enough sample. Like many patients, I had heard only what I had wanted to hear. In my mind I did not have cancer yet. A lot of patients walk around going through the motions but remain convinced that they are not sick. I definitely fell into this category.

I told her about the tests that Dr. Brooks had ordered, and she approved. This was one of the many times that talking to

Dr. Roeder eased my fears. When I asked if she would perform the surgery, she assured me that she would. She hesitantly informed me that I would have to make arrangements for transportation since I would not be able to drive myself home. After reminding me to show up for "prep" Wednesday morning, she said good-bye.

It was beginning to hit me that this was serious and that maybe I was in real trouble. I began to really think about my options, including not getting treatment—not going to the bone scan and not going for the surgery sounded pretty good to me. Maybe it would all go away.

As I reread my research study and prepared for the conference call, the colleague I had e-mailed about my condition stopped by to ask me how things were going. I told him that it sounded real and that I was scheduled for the bone scan and for the biopsy. He was very positive and said maybe it would be like his sister's benign tumor . . . and if not, he had a relative who had breast cancer and lived twenty-five more years after her breast was removed. I know that he meant to cheer me up but it all sounded like so many words.

I gathered my papers and went to my research partner's office. We talked for a few minutes about my diagnosis and then went to work. The conference call went well. The consultant liked my proposal and agreed to work with us on it. She would serve as our statistical advisor. Immediately after concluding the call, my colleague turned to me and said, "You don't have to take it out on her because you're angry about your cancer diagnosis." I was dumbfounded. I felt miserable and misunderstood and guilty for not, according to him, being nice to this woman. I went back to my office and felt terrible. I did not know what felt worse: offending my colleague, not being understood, having to do all the diagnostic tests for a disease that I was terrified of, or being afraid that people were about to discover that I was a bad person. I thought about the most debilitated of the patients I had seen in the past fifteen years. Would I have such an awful and lonely death? All I knew was that I felt horrible and really wanted to die. How was I going to hold my head up?

I called my friend Kathie and asked her if she could pick me up at seven on Wednesday morning to take me to the

Ambulatory Surgery Center at TMC. She said it would not be a problem. Then I called my colleague Jim, who taught at the university, and asked if he could pick me up at half past eleven, after the surgery. Not a problem. He knew where the hospital was because his elderly parents spent a lot of time there.

Home Alone

After several more hours of phone calls, working on my proposal, and seeing clients, I called it a day. I was exhausted and knew that tomorrow would be grueling. At eight the next morning I would get a radioactive isotope injected into my system and then go to visit my psychologist before returning for the bone scan. The radioactive isotope is a tracer element, which allows anything in the bone to appear on the scan. Many patients are initially frightened about having a radioactive substance injected into them, but it is a minute amount and is usually harmless. I was emotionally bewildered but intellectually very clear about what was happening to me.

In the shower I looked at the big breast. I wondered how and why it had gotten that way. I desperately hoped that there was nothing wrong with it, even though it was heavy, painful, and didn't fit in my bra anymore. My long,

The past decade has seen a groundswell of support for research, health care, and reform on behalf of cancer survivors. The National Coalition for Cancer Survivorship provides opportunities and resources for cancer patients to reestablish a normal life during and after their diagnosis and treatment. From the first NCCS Assembly in 1986 until the First National Congress on Cancer Survivorship in 1995, cancer survivors and national spokespeople have donated their time and expertise to the cancer survivorship movement. The NCCS recommends a "single payer" plan for health reform. Such a plan would include a national health program with a consistent approach to the purchase of services, finances, and health care, yet maintain consumer choice of physicians and hospitals.

black hair seemed more precious than ever, as I thought about losing it. I did not like to think of myself as sick. I dreaded having the symptoms that I had read about and witnessed as a psychologist specializing in chronically ill patients. I never wanted to be "one of them." Despite all my professional experience, I was as scared as anyone of being seriously ill.

That night my sleep was troubled by dreams that reminded me of other times when I had been afraid, defenseless, and vulnerable. I dreamed of running into cars and being hit by undetectable objects as I ran at a feverish pace. I would wake up and remind myself that I was at home in bed with Vivi and we were fine. Even though the house was room temperature I was freezing. Wrapped in my nice down comforter, I should have been really cozy, but I had the chills.

Chapter Three

Haven't I Suffered Enough?

Sometimes it is easier to think about dying than to consider the difficulty of continuing to live. I was tired of fighting battles at every juncture of my life. Now as I neared retirement, I was faced with the most arduous battle of all. After the bone scan and biopsy, would it be worth the effort to go on?

Bone Scan

Monday morning finally arrived. The package deal for treatment included navigating new parking lots and offices. I read signs as I drove through the hospital parking lot, taking note of the turn to the Ambulatory Surgery Center as I went. I found my way pretty easily to the Center where I was scheduled at the nuclear medicine department for the bone scan. I checked into the hospital and a plastic band was clamped around my wrist. It seemed like someone now owned me, or worse yet, they might actually lose me! I thought about the implications of this while I received my shot of radioactive isotope and left to see my psychologist.

Therapy was difficult. My psychologist did not know what to say and I did not particularly want to talk about

As a therapist, I realize more than ever the importance of "staying with" the patient. The ambiguity of feelings that clients present to me is always surprising. They do not want to deal with anything, yet want to deal with everything. Now I know how mentally immobilized the patient becomes at this point. If I have not yet established good rapport with the client, I often suggest a spectrum of feelings for them to react to, even if it's just by nodding or head shaking, or being angry and saying "you don't understand how I feel." There is no good reason to get in an argument about intensity of feelings or depth of understanding. As a psychologist, I know it is better to say, "I am distressed or distracted or anxious or worried along with you and I am so glad to be here to be able to share this with you." The "thank you for sharing" phrase may sound trite, but indeed we should be thankful for sharing. It is essential to healing.

anything. Nothing seemed significant. So, I talked about the suddenness of the tests.

"Alice, are you scared?" he asked.

"Yes, a little bit," I admitted.

I talked about how much I liked and trusted the surgeon and gave my assessment of the other doctors. My psychologist pointed out that Dr. Roeder was known for her caring and warmth toward her patients and that's what I was responding to. I agreed. I felt that way about him also.

As the hour drew to a close, I looked down at my hand and realized that I was still wearing my favorite ring. I removed the ring and handed it to him.

"Here, please keep this for me. I cannot wear it for the bone scan and biopsy," I said.

"Sure, I'll keep it and return it to you next week at your appointment. I'll be thinking about you, Alice, and wishing you well."

I guess I was asking him to keep a piece of me, although at the time I thought I was just concerned about keeping my ring safe. My friend Robert, who made the ring, was supposed to visit in a few weeks and I did not want to risk losing it. I also knew that if anything happened to me, my psychologist could use the ring as payment for anything I owed him. Of course, I knew that he would not keep the ring, but would give it to one of my close family members. Since he had been my therapist for a while, he was well acquainted with my family dynamics. He had a lot of history with which to gauge my reactions to any given situation. As a patient just beginning to confront the specter of cancer, I appreciated that my therapist didn't get bogged down in analytical interpretation. Rather, he was as generous as possible in responding to my needs and requests. I did the analytic part all by myself at a later time anyway. The message of caring and honoring my wishes was one that I desperately needed to hear at that time. I wanted him to hug me but I knew that he could not, because of professional boundaries. I knew and felt that he cared about me. But he was a busy man and I was not the center of his life. I felt terribly lonely. If only there were someone that I could turn to. Yet had there been someone there I was not sure what I would discuss with them. Nothing was definite.

I returned to the center at eleven for the bone scan, fifteen minutes early. The waiting room was small and crowded with patients watching TV as they waited for their scans. I wanted to work but it was too noisy to concentrate. I was very nervous and kept thinking, "I don't look sick, so why am I here?" I felt guilty for taking a chair from someone who might really need it. The wait seemed interminable. Finally, I had to go to the bathroom. When I returned, I discovered that in the two minutes I was gone they had called my name. Since I was not present, they had taken another patient. Needless to say, I was unhappy and irritated. I realized that I was getting grumpy. "Lighten up," I told myself, but I was angry and agitated.

After about ten more minutes, a technician led me into an exam room and instructed me to change into a hospital gown. Next, I was asked to lie down on a metal tray coated with a very smooth and shiny porcelain enamel. Then they slowly programmed the camera so that it would automatically adjust to the same distance as it traversed the length of my body. The picture was to extend from the top of my head to my toes. The moving camera seemed to take forever, and then it malfunctioned and stopped at my knees, so they had to repeat the scan on the lower half of my body. After a while, lying still was not much of a problem, as I dozed to the quiet clicking of the

Bone scans are a procedure often ordered for patients with progressed stages of breast cancers. It is also good for anyone with the initial diagnosis to establish a baseline bone scan for future reference. This test is used to determine if the cancer has spread to the bones or if there is other bone disease or bone trauma. You are injected with a phosphonate compound that is radioactive, but almost always harmless. You are then asked to wait between one and five hours and are only allowed to drink fluids. After this, the bones are photographed by a nuclear technician using a gamma camera. The camera scans the body while you lay clothed on a hard table or bed. The procedure lasts from fifteen minutes to one hour.

machine. The process was quiet and did not require going into a tunnel like some CAT scans or MRIs. It took about an hour.

I got dressed and examined the scan. It looked like the picture of a skeleton from an anatomy classroom or physiology laboratory. It was in two parts because of the machine breakdown. To my untrained eye, it looked free from irregularities and strange spots. I was comforted by my unsophisticated assessment, and left feeling much better. I could see where I had a little extra calcium, or so I thought anyway.

I knew better than to ask the technician for results. They are not supposed to say anything but sometimes do so with uncertainty. Many of my clients have had strange experiences from misunderstanding the technician's comments. Because this is likely to happen, technicians are instructed not to give opinions about the results. Since patients are hypervigilant, being told anything other than "you will be called by your physician" can produce undue stress. Of course, waiting for a physician to call is not easy, either. Most physicians are willing to call, or have their nurse call, within twenty-four hours. If they do not get back to the patient by then, she can always call to see when the results will be available.

I stopped to pick up my dog and then went to work for the afternoon. I needed to stay focused so that I did not become overwhelmed with worry about the biopsy on Wednesday. I worked hard and avoided talking about it. This is a time when it is actually quite helpful to focus on other

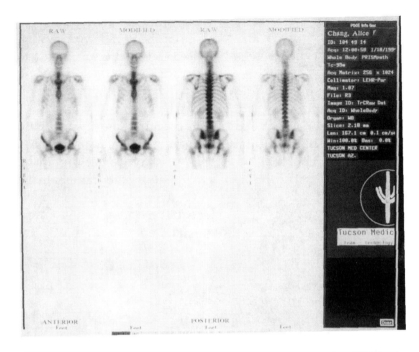

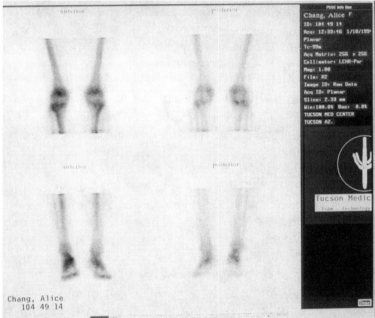

Bone scan

things in life. It is an example of my golden rule of therapy in action: "If you can do something about it, do it. If you can't, let it go for now and do something else." Fortunately, I was in the habit of trying to practice what I preached, and work seemed like the best thing to turn to. I had coped with struggles throughout my life by immersing myself in my work.

Not allowing my condition to consume me was essential. Continuing to work with my colleagues was very important to me, even though I was soon going to have some diminished capacity. That prospect was scary, but would not make me quit. For those whose self-worth is invested in doing or performing, this can be a very anxious and mood-affecting time.

On Tuesday night I did not get much rest. I woke up almost every hour to make sure that I was not late.

Biopsy

Kathie picked me up promptly to take me to the center. I checked in again and got another couple of wristbands, one that indicated my allergies and one for identification. Then the confusion began. They asked if I had had a chest X-ray and if I had blood work. "Yes." Then they asked where and when the tests were completed. "The Cancer Care Center." They eventually found my blood work, but said that they only had a blood count. I insisted that the order had been for total clinical studies, to which they asked me how many vials of blood had been drawn. I told them three and they found the rest of the report. We talked about where and when my chest X-rays had been taken. When I had the chest X-rays there was some confusion because there was another patient named Alice Chang. I told them to look under Alice F. Chang. It was starting to seem like a not-so-funny comedy of errors. Eventually they found them. Both the reports for the blood work and X-rays were normal. A nurse took me in to prepare for surgery.

I was taken into a little room in which there was a comfortable gurney with a basket on a shelf under the bed. I was instructed to undress down to my underwear and put my clothes in the basket. I changed into yet another one of those awful gray gowns.

"What do you do if someone forgets to remove jewelry?" I asked.

"Oh, we tape rings to the patient's fingers so that they won't come off," she replied.

I was glad that I had placed my ring in safekeeping and reminded myself to get it appraised and insured as soon as I could afford to do so. Then the nurse covered me up with a nice warm flannel sheet and took my blood pressure before leaving.

A few minutes later the anesthesiologist showed up and introduced himself. He remarked about my good veins as he was preparing me for the IV tube. Dr. Roeder came in and we talked. We each commented on how the other looked different in this setting and she explained what she was going to do. She informed me that occasionally during a "slice" biopsy, the cells spill and the wound does not heal, although it had never happened to her. What was I supposed to say, "I'm out of here," with the anesthesiologist digging in my hand? So I said, "Well, I guess I just have to trust you and hope for the best, right?" She kept talking to me and I felt safe in her presence.

After a while my hand began to hurt where the anesthesiologist was digging, and when I looked, it was dripping with blood. I reminded him that for every poke there would be a scar, and he said that my veins moved too much. I asked him to find another place on my arm. Dr. Roeder left for the operating room. The anesthesiologist put the IV in a larger vein at the crook of my elbow. His supervisor came in, examined the IV, and introduced himself.

Then they wheeled me into the operating room where I could see my surgeon sitting at a little table with her back to me. They slid me onto the operating table and before I knew it the anesthesia was going into my veins. They joked about my being too knowledgeable as they clamped a device to my finger that would measure oxygen volume throughout the surgery. I was pleased with their state-of-the-art equipment. When I asked if they were going to intubate me, I was told I would receive a mask instead. I joked with them about wanting to keep the caps on my four front teeth. I could tell the surgeon was laughing and everyone was feeling confident.

Recovery

Suddenly I was in the recovery room and I was cold and shiv-ering. Someone put warm flannel blankets on me and I could hear them talking about my blood pressure. I opened my eyes and Dr. Roeder was leaning over my gurney at the foot of the bed: "Hi. You did really well. I made a little incision about an inch and a half long." She showed me by parting her thumb and forefinger. I am sure she was hoping I would not exagger-ate the size of the cut by the gauze packing on top of my chest. "The best thing for pain is to use ice for the first twenty-four hours."

"Fine," I said. I had learned to do the "fine" bit from her. That is what she would say when she did not want to agree but knew that someone was right. I didn't particularly want to take any more advice from doctors, even if it was to my benefit.

"Do you need any pain medication, Alice?"

"I don't think so. I've never used any when it's been given to me."

"I did a really neat job and took two slices off the crown of the tumor," Dr. Roeder said.

"Fibroid, right?" I checked.

"No, Alice, tumor. It's a tumor."

I still did not believe her. "No," I said, "not a tumor."

She nodded her head. "Yes, a tumor.

"The slices have been sent to pathology and we'll have the results tomorrow. You can call me. Are there any family mem-bers or friends waiting for you that you'd like me to talk to?"

"Nope," I said. "No one."

Someone asked about how I was getting home. I told them a colleague was picking me up since I did not want to get arrested for "drunk walking" and I had already been told that I would not be allowed to drive out of the parking lot. Other-wise, I would have walked home since it was only three miles. I told Dr. Roeder that I had an appointment with Dr. Brooks. "Good," she replied.

After Dr. Roeder left, the nurses said something about treating my high blood pressure. "No treatment for high blood pressure," I replied. "It's not covered by my insurance. It was exempted for two years from my policy." The charge nurse informed me that my blood pressure was 140 over 120. "Too bad," I answered. "This is part of a surgery recovery period and not hypertension," she responded. "Okay," I said. They broke a capsule of medicine and put it under my tongue.

I began to feel well enough to sit up, or so I thought. I became immediately nauseated and dizzy, so I lay back down. My blood pressure had rapidly dropped. I heard someone say that my ride had arrived and they told him to wait. I could not even get up and felt terrible for inconveniencing Jim. Kindly, he assured me that he had time to wait.

The nurses read some written instructions about after-surgery wound care to me. They ordered some pain medication. I got dressed and headed for the hospital exit where Jim would be waiting for me. They wanted to put me in a wheelchair but I refused. I wanted my computer, which I had been using before surgery, and a nurse offered to carry it for me. She said that I should not carry anything for a day or two.

I was a bit groggy and thankful that I didn't have to walk the three miles. Jim took me home and I went straight to bed. An hour or so later I woke up and got some ice in a plastic bag with a towel wrapped around it. The cold eased the pain and I fell asleep. I woke up again and put the bag in the freezer, and then returned to sleep. I remember repeating the sequence several times and the next morning I woke up feeling okay.

Thursday morning I went to work as usual. In the last week I had been through more than I wanted to think about. So I picked up my mail and went to the office. I was a little slow and had some pain, but it was tolerable. I thought about how my patients had complained of pain and how little I had experienced, so far. How much of the pain experience after this surgery was psychological and how much was physiological, I wondered. Over the years I had taught pain management to so many of my clients and I wondered if it would work in my case also. Tolerating pain, both physical and emotional, was a skill I had honed throughout my life. I had not heard of other surgeons recommending the ice bag routine. "Too bad," I thought. It occurred to me that a little manual on postsurgical care would be really helpful.

I missed my surgeon already and felt foolish for being so attached when I didn't really know her that well. But she seemed to care so much and I, like all patients, needed that more at this time than any other in my life. She was a good doctor and she had been open and honest with me. It was so refreshing to feel as though my doctor was treating me with respect and caring. This was not a common trait in the physicians whom I had consulted on both a personal and professional basis. When I did see these qualities in those who sent me referrals, I was delighted. Whether they were colleagues or patients, I tried to emphasize the importance of this to the physicians I knew.

Waiting

By noon on Thursday, I was beginning to get anxious. I called my psychologist and left word that I wanted to talk with him and that I had an appointment with the oncologist that day. I thought it was his birthday and did not want to bother him, but I reminded myself that he had called earlier when I was not home. I tried to work, but it was futile. Later I realized that I was mistaken about his birthday.

I sent an e-mail to my brother, George, who knew that I was going through all of these procedures. I had shared my reflections and feelings about what I was going through with him and asked that he not discuss my situation with other family members. George and I had developed a closeness in our adult years that we had not shared in childhood. Growing up, he was clearly my parents' favorite. While it often seemed like I could do no right, he was the prized son who could do no wrong. As adults we had worked hard on our relationship, and had been rewarded with an enduring trust and lasting friendship. Considering our rocky start, we both realize how exceptional this is.

Then the hunt began. I called Dr. Brooks' office to see if he had received the pathology report from the biopsy. His nurse called back to tell me that they had not. I could not concentrate on anything else at this point. I called Dr. Roeder's office. They had not received the report, either. They called the pathology office and were told that they would have the report by four. I insisted that I could not wait that long, that I had to see Dr. Brooks and didn't want to hear the news from him. Dr. Roeder had won me over with her caring bedside manner, and I would be much more comfortable discussing the findings with her. Jean said that they would call if they got any news. I continued to be very anxious and could not focus my mind or do any work.

If I really had cancer, did I want to go through all of this aggravation? How sick was I, really? And did I want to suffer anymore? I had suffered enough from life, from childhood, through a career. I was not responsible to anyone and no one in the family really knew anything. I did not think anyone would care, anyway. I was a worthless person that no one really cared for or respected. I was an unaccomplished girl, not a real scientist. In my overachieving family, I could not even be considered truly successful. I could still just find out what my life expectancy would be, and refuse treatment.

At precisely three twenty-seven, the phone rang: "Hi Alice, this is Vanessa Roeder calling. Jean said you called about the results from the pathology folks."

"Yes, I did."

She said those horrible words again: malignant tumor. I gasped, "Oh, not benign, and not a fibroid, huh?"

"Nope, and I know what things must be going through your head."

We talked and she told me about some patients who had done really well after treatment. She talked about a fast-growing cancer, and about the other sample going for hormone receptor tests and waiting for another week to see those test results. She said that we needed to do chemotherapy, and then a mastectomy, and then radiation.

"How big is the tumor?" I asked. Dr. Roeder hedged and said that she did not like to say because she could never know how much was inflammation and how much was real tumor, but it was probably about two and a half inches in diameter. A sample of my breast skin tissue revealed that it was in the skin also. She told me that it was important for me to get treatment and that this was the best regimen. Follow the treatment plan and trust them, was her suggestion. Then she asked about making an appointment for the next week to have my stitches removed. "No," I said. I would call later.

I asked if I would be grossed out when I took the dressing off my wound that night. Many of my patients had been very upset about their scars from the biopsy. The surgeon does not have to be too careful or neat about sewing up the wound, especially if the plan is for a mastectomy. Many surgeons hurriedly close the wound to minimize blood loss. However, a skilled surgeon can close the wound neatly and still keep blood loss to a minimum. A neat wound means more thoughtfulness and understanding of the patient's feelings. This is the last time the patient will see her former breast. It is easier if the scar is neat.

"I think I did a very neat job on you and you won't be grossed out. If it upsets you, call and yell at me." Dr. Roeder laughed. "I mean it!" Then she said, "You will go and start treatment, won't you?" I said, "Yeah, sure." She hung up and I headed out to my appointment with Dr. Brooks feeling comforted by our conversation.

A Good Time to Die

Then I was driving to the Cancer Care Center where I would again be told by a very bright, proper doctor that I had cancer. What could I do next? Well, I would hear about the real treatment options and have time to consider them. Would I want to do drug trials and be a guinea pig? I could die in the name of science and make some meaningful contribution of my life. By the time I had driven the six miles or so to the center, I was back to feeling worthless. Leaving my dog in the car, I headed for Dr. Brooks' office. Walking the few feet from the elevator to the office door felt like walking ten miles. When I entered his office someone said, "Hi, Alice, we got all of your reports."

I said, "I know," and sat down in the large, well-lit waiting room. The support staff for five oncologists were talking on phones, laughing and talking together, or looking at patients. The room seemed huge with an open reception area and only a half wall with a window separating it from the work area. As the staff discussed patients with each other and on the phone, it seemed like a too public display of something that should have been private. Other patients took all of the corner spots so I could not find a place to hide. I sat in the middle wishing for some privacy while I looked at books and magazines.

I was called into the inner office by a nurse who took my weight and blood pressure. Dr. Brooks came in and started talking about cancer treatment. He was very direct and explained everything that I had previously heard about. "We're going to give you 5 FU (5-Fluorouracil), Adriamycin (Doxorubicin), and Cytoxan (Cyclophosphamide) and you'll lose your hair. You read the books on chemotherapy. You're going to vomit and you're going to feel nauseated, but we'll give you drugs to control those reactions." I asked him about the individual drugs and he assured me that I would not have any side effects that would prohibit me from continuing my day-to-day activities. I am sure he wanted to give me the most positive of all possible worlds but it sure sounded like wishful thinking. The more he talked, the more I did not want to go through with treatment. I was beginning to feel more comfortable with the idea of dying.

I asked the doctor about clinical trials and he explained that they happened to be doing a Stage Three clinical trial on an antiemetic drug. They could put me into one of three categories ranging from no drug to adequate dosage. One advantage of being in the drug study was that they sent a nurse home with the patient for the first twenty-four hours, in case there might be any severe reactions. That was very appealing, since I lived alone and did not want to be a burden to anyone. I told him that I was interested in the cause of science, and

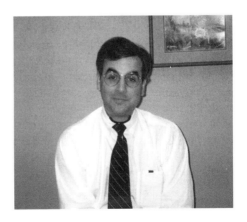

Dr. Brooks

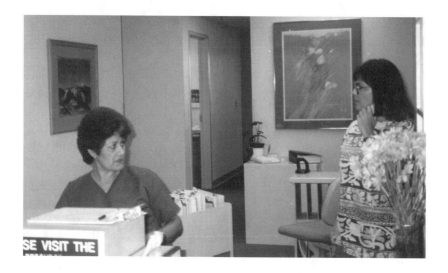

Dr. Brooks' receptionist Rose, and Vicki

asked for a copy of all of my reports. He was ready to start me on chemotherapy treatments then and there.

I did not speak, and finally shrugged my shoulders at him.

Dr. Brooks looked at me quizzically and said, "You aren't thinking about anything besides getting treated, are you?"

I said that I was, and he asked what I was thinking. I said: "Well, I have had a good life, yet a hard life of struggles and I don't want to struggle anymore. This is a good time for me to die. I am semiretired and unencumbered since I don't have clients. I have no outside obligations and I'm not even sure that I can pay my medical bills. I have accomplished a lot in life. I have done a lot of good for a lot of people, and I feel very comfortable about dying. I am not sure that I want to have treatment." The look on his face was one of disgust and disbelief. He said, "Of course it is up to you."

He asked about my medical insurance and kept telling me not to worry about the medical bills, at least the ones associated with him. He had the nurse who was working on the experimental drug studies explain them to me. I asked her a lot of questions and she explained the protocols in detail. I took a copy of everything she had. She was also told to give me a copy of the records that I had requested. I asked her a bunch of questions about hair loss, diet, reactions, fatigue, and so on. She was very thorough and calmly answered all of them.

While scanning the office, my eyes stopped at the area where I would receive the chemotherapy treatment—if I agreed to it. An image of cattle lined up for slaughter flashed across my mind. There was a nurse's station in the middle, with a row of chairs on either side of the room. The brown imitation-leather chairs had wide wooden armrests. Above each chair was a chain hanging from a little rail on the ceiling, which circled about twelve inches around each chair. The bags of liquid chemicals were hung from the chains while patients received an IV drip. If anyone accompanied the patient, they sat on a hassock or in the next treatment chair. Everyone sat with their back to the wall facing the center of the room. As people drifted by it seemed as if the patient was nothing more than a chair with a drip bag that occasionally had to be replaced. Curtains hung on ceiling tracks could have formed room dividers but they were left open instead. There was no privacy. I didn't like it. I left.

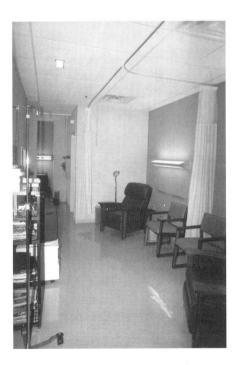

Treatment rooms

Chapter Four

Chemotherapy

Like a handful of dice, treatment options were quickly rolled out in front of me. If I took the chemotherapy, would it offer me enough quality of life to balance the wrenching side effects? How would I cope with hair loss and an emerging new identity?

This Is a Bad Dream

I left Dr. Brook's office on Thursday horrified by the specter of my own future. I was in a state of shock. Seeing Vivi asleep in the front seat of my car roused me from my dread and gave me a moment of happiness. I told her that if I died she would go back to Kansas City and live with our friends, Peggy and Walt. At the sound of their names she got up and started looking for them. She wagged her tail and bounced from window to window as I drove the three miles home. Sadness settled over me as I thought about the merits of living versus dying.

When we arrived home Vivi ran in the yard for a while and I wandered mechanically through the rooms of my small house: the kitchen, the bathroom, the guest bedroom, the family room, the living room, my bedroom. The sun was starting to set when I finally looked at the treatment guidelines Dr. Brooks had given me. I could not understand much of it. I kept thinking about my clients who had died and all the mixed emotions I had about each one's slow and sometimes painful death. The fact that not every cancer patient has lots of pain was overshadowed by my fear. I was not afraid of dying, but my courage dwindled as I dwelled on the possibility of pain.

I also remembered that cancer patients often don't die of cancer as much as from a compromised immune system. They are sometimes attacked by another disease while they slowly deteriorate from the effects of cancer. In the cases I had seen, the lingering nature of the disease sometimes bought the family more time to grieve, but they also suffered as they worked through issues during this period. I suspected that my family wouldn't care so much, and might even resent being bothered with my death. I thought about my power of attorney for medical and financial decisions, which I had completed in 1992, when I had revised my will. Thank goodness, one less thing to worry about.

I did not want to have cancer and certainly did not want to go through all the complications that I had witnessed others experience. To top it off, my cancer sounded worse than any of the other cases I had seen or heard about. My clients had not received chemotherapy until they were definitely terminal—I later learned that the earlier treatment protocols were different and less effective than current ones. They underwent surgery and radiation first. I was haunted by the image of my friend from graduate school who had a throat tumor. He had undergone surgery the day after diagnosis and then was radiated until his neck and the side of his head turned purple with burns and his voice became hoarse.

I still felt like I was in a good place to let go. I had served a lot of people and accomplished many things. That I would be missed by anyone seemed unlikely and I didn't particularly want to struggle anymore. The past year had been a mixed bag of successes and failures. Even though other people disagreed, I saw myself as a failure, overall. They did not know how much I wanted to quit, since I always kept a full stable of projects and plans. Recently I had proposed new research, ran for two leadership positions in the American Psychological Association, and one in the Asian-American Psychological Association. Much to my surprise, I won all three. I was receiving validation and encouragement from my peers whom I had always thought of as being in the inner circle, while I hovered around the edges of it. I thought about how much I liked my surgeon and how she seemed to understand how I felt—something I had only experienced with my psychologist. I also thought about all of the things that I was ashamed of and that if I died, would die with me, especially if I destroyed all the letters, journals, and logs that I had kept for the last thirty years. Then I realized that I was not ready to destroy them, yet.

Finally, I pulled myself away from the scoreboard of my life, and decided to call Jay, my former physician and friend in Kansas City. I had faxed him all of the reports and wanted to pour over every detail of them. As an oncologist and friend he was invaluable to me at this time. Because he was not in when I called, I left a message with his daughter. All I could do was nurse my mixed emotions while I waited for his call.

I knew that I was not well. The painful breast lump and sharp chest pains I was now experiencing would not let me forget that. Dr. Roeder had warned me that pressure from the tumor could cause chest pain. I wanted to talk with her again, even though we had just spoken a few hours earlier. My fear rendered me incapable of making a decision. I was going to begin chemotherapy, but backed out because I couldn't deal with it. I was going to volunteer for drug trials, but changed my mind after reading through the protocols at home. The best thing for me would be if I

The concept of "face" is ambiguous. It can mean bringing pride or shame primarily to the family, but to others as well. Someone diagnosed with a chronic or terminal illness has called attention to her problems, and therefore risks bringing shame and embarrassment to her family. The patient may struggle with saving face in the family and the double bind of whether to further comply with a physician or psychologist, whose "face" will be disgraced if she discontinues treatment. In my own practice I try to reframe issues to accommodate my clients' cultural predispositions. If, for example, I am working with an Asian family concerned about saving face, I would say something such as, "This surgery will help your daughter continue her educational achievements and filial obligations."

could die quickly and not tell anyone anything. This would "save face" for everyone concerned. I would also save everyone a lot of money. How was I going to pay for this anyway?

Decisions, Decisions, Decisions

Decision making happens at every juncture of the cancer story. The first one I had to make was whether or not to get treatment. My knee-jerk reaction was to refuse it. I had moved to Tucson to rest and eventually die. Maybe "eventually" would come sooner than I thought. It was time to make some critical decisions. Usually if a patient gets a lumpectomy, she is not going to have a mastectomy. Radiation without chemotherapy typically follows. Lumpectomy is a viable option if the tumor is small and/or the lump has well-defined margins with encapsulated growth, and if there is no evidence of cancer elsewhere. As much as I wished this were an option for me, it wasn't. An aggressive protocol scared me to death because so much medication is required. I knew what would happen: my hair would fall out, I would get sick, I wouldn't feel like eating. Over the years, I had urged my clients to get the most suitable treatment for their illness. Now I was in their shoes.

Friends in the Business

After seeing the oncologist, I received a series of phone calls, starting with Dr. Bidwell, a friend and former colleague. He knew about my predicament and was calling to see what the biopsy results were. "It's definite," I told him. "I have cancer." We talked about the clinical trial for the new antiemetic drug. It was in phase three of the FDA cycle. He had heard about the drug and thought it was well on its way to being approved.

I told him that I was not sure if I wanted to be treated. "Alice, that does not necessarily have to mean the end of your life," he responded. "My mother had a tumor and didn't have surgery. She had a spontaneous remission and is still alive at the ripe old age of ninety. I would rather see you have a better chance of being an old lady some day, but it's up to you." We both knew how rare spontaneous remission is. It almost never happens and a patient is unwise to expect it. "Okay," I said, and thanked him. He told me he would call again, if I didn't mind. Not really caring, I said the polite thing, "Sure." I did not want to cause anyone more problems.

Then the phone rang again and it was Amie, the daughter of my good friends Robert and Dee. Amie and I are very close and she needed to talk to someone about her divorce. After discussing this for a while, she asked, "How are you doing and what's going on in your life?" I answered that I was not well and that I had just come from the doctor's office with a positive diagnosis for cancer of the left breast. I told her I was trying to decide what to do with the options and treatment plans before me and that I could not see myself as sick. "Oh," Amie gasped, "I'm so embarrassed at going on and on about the trivial things in my life when something really serious is happening with you!" I told her that her situation was important too, and we laughed and talked for a little bit longer. When I hung up, I knew that we both felt better.

As the evening passed however, I felt nauseated and faint. So I went to bed, even though it was not quite eight. I was used to sleeping when I felt depressed or sick. In bed, I read the reports over and over again, wondering if the information they conveyed could really be true. How would I tell my family?

After I had been dozing and waking every few minutes for an hour and a half, the phone rang. I was relieved to hear Jay's voice. He is one of those doctors whose strong, velvety voice exudes patience and understanding. "Hi, Jay. How are you? How are your kids?" I also asked about his mother-in-law, who is a good friend of mine. Jay asked about the proposed treatment regimen and I explained the chemotherapy and clinical trials for the antiemetic drug. When I told him that I did not understand everything on the report, he had me read it to him, line by line, while he interpreted it: "This is a positive reading of a very aggressive cancer and it needs to be treated aggressively," Jay declared. He asked me about treatment again and I informed him that Dr. Brooks had wanted me to start on chemotherapy that day and that we had discussed clinical trials. I told him how I explained my willingness to die and that the oncologist had said that it was "up to me" and walked out. Jay chided me for even considering anything other than treatment. He said that Dr. Brooks was probably upset by my ambivalence. This was hard for me to believe because I couldn't see why anyone would want to save my life.

I asked Jay about the chemicals used in treatment and he explained each one in detail. Then he said, "Go and get treatment, Alice. No clinical trials. They may look good now but you don't know three or four years down the line what it could mean to your health. Use what's tried and true." He recommended Zofran for the nausea, and said that they would give it to me as I got ready to start the chemotherapy.

We discussed hair loss. The bad news was that I would lose all of my hair. The good news was that the insurance company would pay for a wig, or I could call the American Cancer Society and they would loan me one. But the hair would grow back. We also talked about how food might taste differently because of the chemicals. Since reading the literature from the oncologist's office, I had lots of questions. "You know you're really sick, don't you?" Jay said. "Oh, no, I'm not sick at all," I answered. Then we discussed all of the patients that he had referred to me over the years. "I know," Jay said, "that's the point. We need you. There aren't many people like you." A part of me said, "So?" Another part of me enjoyed the pat on the back. Then I said something I have commonly heard from cancer patients, "My oncologist hates me. He won't see me anymore. I can't go back and get treated." This is a reaction that many people have after disagreeing with their doctor. They are scared to go back and change their minds.

So my smart, seasoned oncologist friend said, "Well, we all miss you. You and the dog get on a plane tomorrow, come to Kansas City and stay with my mother-in-law. I'll treat you. You know she has an extra room and you are welcome to stay, I'm sure." Well, now I was really embarrassed. Here was my friend selflessly offering his help, when I couldn't even decide if my life was worth saving. So I said, "Oh, I will call about treatment."

By the end of our two-hour conversation I had decided to get treatment. The next day, January 20, I started six cycles of chemotherapy at twenty-one-day intervals.

My doctor recommended a six-cycle chemotherapy regimen for my aggressive breast cancer. Each of the six treatments consisted of three different chemotherapy drugs and premedication to prevent nausea and vomiting. The drugs are 5-FU, Adriamcycin, and Cytoxan. The antinausea regimen consists of a combination of Zofran and Decadron.

Chemotherapy Begins

I went to Dr. Brook's office and received my chemical cocktail by IV drip. I was so scared that I got the chills, so they covered me up with a very cozy homemade afghan. The antiemetic Zofran was administered first and felt cold as it went in. Luckily, it was only a small amount and didn't take long. In truth, I was more afraid of being nauseated and vomiting than I really was nauseated. In fact I was not nauseated at all during the chemical drip. I sat in the "cattle room" along the wall with others who appeared to be more calm than I as they read

Undergoing chemotherapy treatments can be lonely and time consuming. There are some simple activities that can be done during treatment to help you relax and boost your spirits. Reading, especially a good novel or even just looking at pictures, can be a fun diversion. If a VCR is available, bring along a movie. Your favorite music can be comforting during this time. Many people find classical music to be particularly relaxing. Writing is very effective for keeping your mind occupied and is a good outlet for expressing feelings. Good old-fashioned conversation is another excellent diversion. Relaxation tapes, whether they offer guided exercises, music, nature sounds, or a combination of all three, can be very helpful. Finally, this is a great time to take up meditation. But be warned: Chemotherapy has a way of adversely conditioning you to certain experiences. I used to love Celtic music. I found it so calming and relaxing that I decided to listen to it during my treatments. Now the once calming sound of Celtic music reawakens all the physical sensations I had during treatment. At the first sound of it, I feel nauseated and scared to death.

magazines and conversed with those around them.

I decided I would use this time to work and soon realized that less demanding tasks, such as typing simple correspondence on my laptop computer, were best suited to this situation. After a few visits, I decided to bring a tape of my favorite music. Because Zofran has a sedative effect, I would doze off for short periods. I was thankful that I only had three miles to drive home and then I could take my antiemetic prescription, Torecan, and go to bed.

This exercise was taught to me in 1976 by Norman Shealy. I modify it to suit my needs, or the needs of my clients.

1. Put yourself in the most comfortable position possible. Uncross your arms and legs and rest your head comfortably. Close your eyes and imagine the sounds in the room getting quieter until they finally fade away. Inhale deeply and say to yourself, "I am." When you exhale say, "relaxed." Say this to yourself slowly, breathing in and out, "I am . . . relaxed."

2. Then visualize or make a picture in your mind of a cancer cell, however you imagine it might look, and surround it with many healthy pink cells until it becomes very small and then vanishes. Think of fresh, clean, healthy cells populating your body. Rest, let the healthy cells take over, and relax.

3. Slowly, let yourself become more alert until you are wide awake, still relaxed, and keeping that positive feeling of control.

A variation of this exercise is to become relaxed with the deep breathing and then to concentrate on letting the pain or nausea go away.

Side Effects of Chemotherapy

The second treatment was not nearly as bad. At least I knew what to expect. I had already begun to lose my hair, and a lot of the anxiety about the procedure itself had abated. I realized that it was not as bad as I anticipated. The first traumatic event after diagnosis is the loss of hair, then the fingernails change color. The nails happen at the same time as the hair loss, but it depends on how fast they grow, because a nail's worth of normal color has to grow out. I have fast-growing nails, so one of the first things that happened in response to the chemotherapy was this discoloration. Every week I noticed more discolored nail growing from the nail bed.

I told my doctor that my fingernails looked like they were dead. They were, and he added, "Usually they don't grow out this fast. The chemotherapy must really be working."

> If my clients have a pet, I try to ensure that they can keep it. A pet usually does not react to hair loss or weight changes. They just continue to be unconditionally loving and accepting. They can be a stabilizing factor in a world that has become topsy-turvy. Sometimes patients are asked to give up their pets for a while if they are going to undergo a bone marrow transplant, and that is really difficult. My miniature greyhound has been with me for eleven years. She was a great comfort to me during my treatments.

I started to become obsessed with them and took a lot of pictures. Earlier in my life, I had been diagnosed with psoriatic arthritis. This caused little ridges to form on my fingernails. Now I had discolored nails with little ridges on them. Great. I indulged in some serious self-pity. However, a nice side effect of the chemotherapy was that the psoriasis cleared from my skin and has been better ever since, although some of it returned a couple of years later. When I learned that many of the chemotherapy medications interrupted the psoriasis, I joked about having chemotherapy every couple of years to help my skin.

Canker sores and lesions in the throat also result from chemotherapy. This happens because the lowered immune system makes you more vulnerable to infection. The doctor gave me what they called "miracle mouthwash," which, when swished and swallowed several times a day, diminished much of the pain from the sores. It is important to have something safe to swallow since the sores can spread throughout the esophagus. "Miracle mouthwash" consists of Benadryl, Nystatin, and other components that shorten the life of the infection. Some people also find it helpful to rinse their mouths with a solution of one-fourth teaspoon baking soda and one-eighth teaspoon salt dissolved in one cup of warm water, followed by a plain water rinse.

Another part of chemotherapy that I had to get used to was regular lab tests. When the results were abnormal, I was upset and would demand answers: "Why are they abnormal? Why is my blood count less? What happened since the last test to cause this?"

Since chemotherapy breaks down the immune system, it is not surprising that some of the results were abnormal. Of course, the doctors kept checking the immune system to see if it was strong enough to handle the next treatment. Sometimes I had a strong enough immune system (a high enough white blood cell count), and sometimes I did not. Once I had to wait an additional week before I received my next chemotherapy treatment. Some patients require an immune system booster, and in some treatment protocols it is standard practice to administer one.

Because chemotherapy can cause nausea, it is common for patients to abstain from eating. During chemotherapy I was told to eat anything I wanted. Everyone agreed that maintaining body weight as much as possible was important. *Slowly* eating whatever you desire can help. It also helps if friends can join you for a leisurely meal. Never underestimate the value of conversation at mealtime. By occupying your mind, you can diminish a lot of the anxiety about vomiting. I found that I ate slower than my friends and often did not finish, but eating became much more tolerable with company. Also, drinking water often results in nausea. Like many patients, I fared better with carbonated drinks. I grew to particularly like fruit-flavored carbonated water.

I had been warned that the inevitable hair loss would take place in three to six weeks. In preparation, I had ordered a wig from a mail-order catalog and, photograph in hand, went to the wig stylist and told him, "Cut it like it is in this photo." I was ready. Then the inevitable happened. One morning while I was taking a shower my long, black hair that I had had for

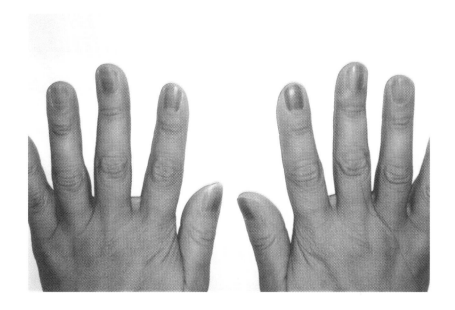

Just as hair cells quickly die from chemotherapy, so do fingernails.

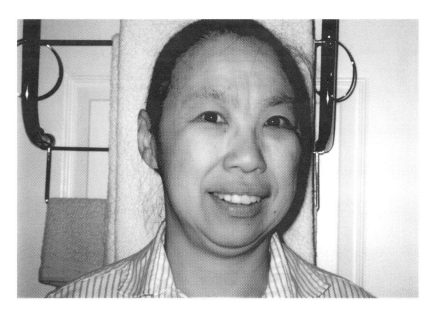

Losing my hair the first time was more traumatic than losing my breast.

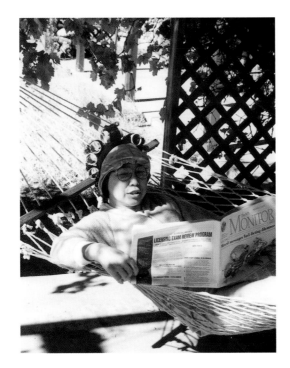

After I lost my hair, a friend sent me some wonderful hairpieces. Here's me and my curlers in the sun.

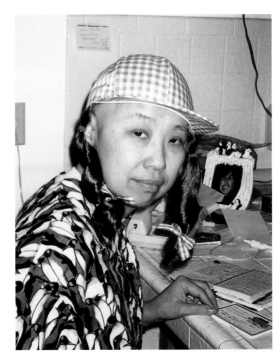

Me in pigtails. Humor was essential during this time.

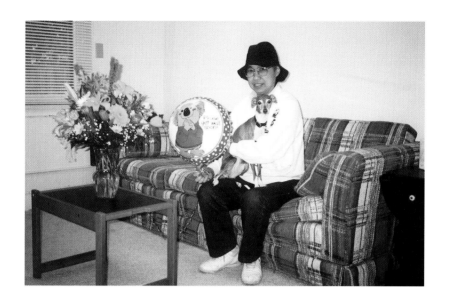

My favorite hat and my best friend.

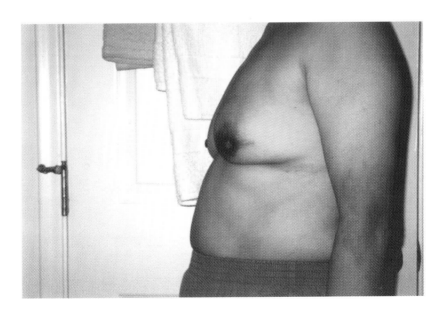

The last night with two breasts.

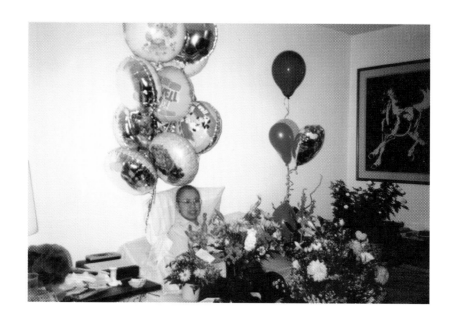

The funeral I staged on my first day home after surgery.

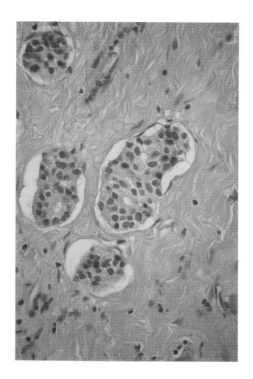

A section of breast tissue that shows nests of malignant cells within the lymphatic vascular space.

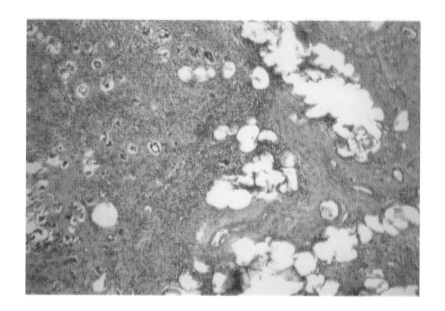

Immature breast cancer cells in the lymphatic tissue.

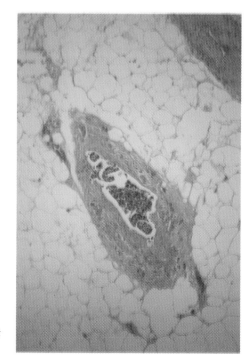

A group of malignant breast cancer cells in fatty tissue.

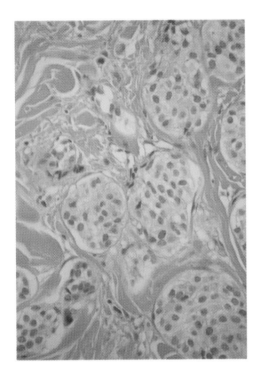

A section of breast tissue that shows multiple nests of neoplasm, or a new growth of abnormal cells.

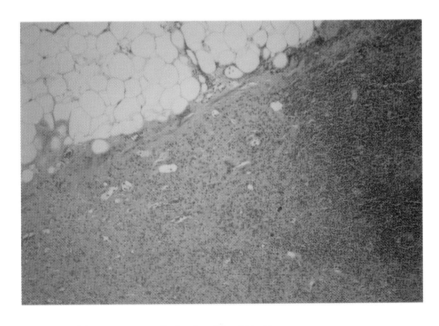

A sea of breast cancer cells bordered by fatty tissue.

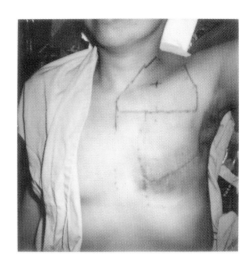

Time to have the radiation
rays concentrated to the
collarbone area.

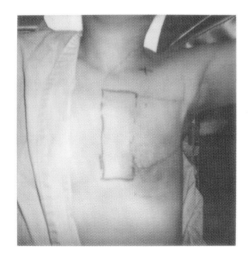

Being mapped for the more
shallow electron rays that
are applied to the sternum.

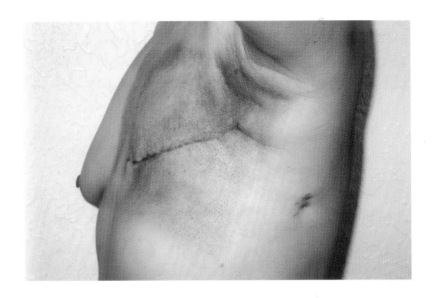

After radiation the burns healed quickly due to conscientious skin care.

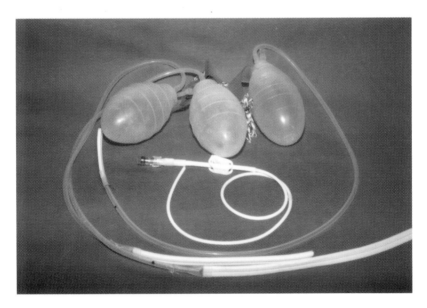

Drain bottles used to remove excess liquid after surgery. The catheter is in the center. The thick, white part was installed in my body.

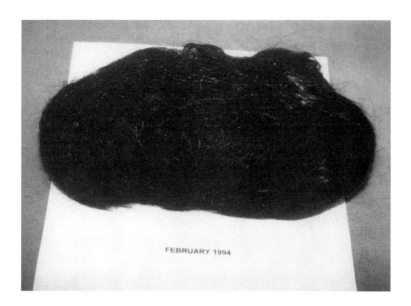

FEBRUARY 1994

Saved Hair

thirty years began to come out by the handful. I carefully saved all my hair, dried it with a towel, and stored it in a plastic bag. I still would not let myself believe that I was sick, just that I was bald and badly traumatized. Those who have not lost their hair, or have not lost their hair suddenly, cannot fully understand the extent of this trauma. This was the first time I lost my hair. Like the chemotherapy treatments, the second time was not as bad.

Cancer forces you to do nurturing things for yourself and to redefine your self-image. I had never worn hats before I got cancer. But I bought a hat before my hair fell out. It was a nice, black, velvet fedora, and it was on sale to boot. Unfortunately, after I lost my hair it was too big for my head. So now I remind my clients to buy hats a size smaller if they shop before hair loss.

I have a favorite hat that has become something like a security blanket. After all this time it's a little worse for the wear but no less valuable to me. When I went for my mastectomy, I informed the doctors and nurses, "You can't take my hat off." Well, I know they took it off, but when I woke up that hat was sitting on my head. Hats are just one way to do something special for yourself.

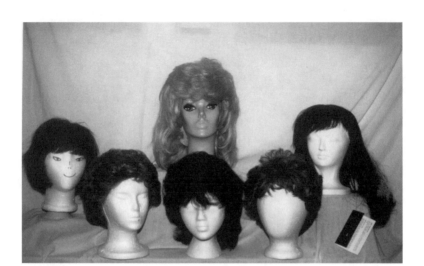

Hairpieces

Hair loss is difficult for the friends of cancer patients because it is a visible reminder that they may lose someone they love. So they can be very rejecting at times. I had friends who said, "Don't come see me. I don't want to see you without your hair." It hurt a lot, but at some point I realized that they were acting like the friends and relatives of some of my former clients. They had their reasons.

And I also had friends who helped make me feel as accepted and valued as ever. The Henions are very spiritual, and artists by profession. Over the years, they had made jewelry for me and often visited after I moved to Tucson. They came to Tucson for the International Gem and Mineral Show about the same time that I lost my hair. Dee gave me a big hug and said, "What a lovely head you have. It's shaped so nice. Don't you think so, Robert?" Robert gave me a hug, rubbed my head, and agreed, adding that now I looked like a Tibetan monk. "Now you're really a mystery," he said. We hugged, laughed, and cried, all at the same time.

I was not sure if my head was well shaped or not, but it felt wonderful to be hugged and to have someone rub my bald head, while telling me that I looked like a Tibetan monk. Having learned this lesson from personal experience, I have encouraged patients' families and friends to support their loved one at this time. Affectionate physical contact and kind words go a long way. When a loved one is in trouble, many people quickly learn to be more demonstrative with their feelings.

In May I traveled to Washington, D.C. to attend the first Behavioral Health Conference on Women, sponsored by the APA. While there, I met Jocelyn Elders, then Surgeon General. I wore my wig, and no one noticed.

My body was becoming pretty important to me. I noticed that I was getting bloated and constipated. So I tried the usual array of products advertised on TV—suppositories, ointments, and Preparation H. Well, sometimes they helped, but most of the time I still had lots of discomfort. Because I was too embarrassed to say anything, I just suffered. Finally, I called Vicki, the nurse at Dr. Brooks' office, and told her that I was having an awful problem. "Well," she said, "that's not so awful. You need to take a stool softener and drink a lot of liquids." I mentioned the names of the products that I had been using and she informed me that they were lubricants not softeners. I felt so stupid. She suggested that I try Senokot, a nonprescription natural softener and laxative derived from the senna plant. I got some and it worked relatively quickly. This was to come in handy over the next year, as I found that constipation was a side effect of many drugs.

While working through hair loss and other cancer issues, your therapist must be accessible. The first thing I say to my

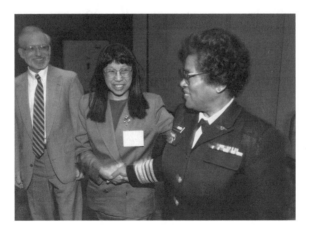

It's hard to tell I'm wearing a wig.

clients is, "Call me when you feel the need. It will be much easier if you call me and we talk for two or three minutes than if you just obsess, worry, or fret about it. So just call. I always return my calls, so know that I will." I will call until I reach them. If I haven't called within twenty-four hours, they have been instructed to call me again in case I didn't receive the message.

Why Me?

"Why Me?" is a question that just about every patient asks. Usually, it is the first question that comes to mind after being diagnosed. In the beginning I had a very harsh answer for myself: I had gotten cancer because I was a lifelong depressive and deserved to have bad things happen to me. I no longer believe that I deserved cancer or that my depressive moods caused it. Fortunately, I had good insurance that paid for psychotherapy. It helps a lot. Support groups also may be helpful. Support groups are good at some times and not at others. After attending a group meeting I have had clients say, "I went to this support group and they said that one out of eight people get breast cancer. Is that so?"

And I said, "That is a statistic that I have heard, but what does it mean to you?"

"That means I'm going to die. At the meeting they told me I am going to die. I don't know if I can go to the meetings." Patients often imagine the worst when hearing statistics like this. As a therapist it is important for me to understand and guide them through these reactions.

Chapter Five

The Drive-Through Mastectomy and Radiation

As surgery drew near, it seemed like I was about to embark on a long journey without knowing what the terrain would be like or where I would eventually find myself. The treatment plan was under way and there was no stopping it! Along the way, I got a crash course in getting support, managing pain, and caring for fluid drains. I also became well-versed in dealing with scars, bone marrow transplants, radiation burns, frozen shoulders, and lymphedema. By June I had completed all six courses of chemotherapy and it was time for surgery to remove my left breast. Although I told myself that I didn't need anybody, I brought my friend Peggy in from Kansas City.

Preparing for Surgery

Two days before surgery I met Peggy at the airport. The next day we took off for a little adventure—a time that I anticipated would be a break from my crisis. We drove to a Native American trading post in Safford, Arizona. On the way home we

I try to help my clients get the support they need. Isolated patients are at risk of immersing themselves in unhealthy environments or habits to relieve their loneliness. I remember a patient who came to see me two years after her second mastectomy. She was by herself for both surgeries, which had been about two years apart. Now she was in her early sixties, alone and depressed. She had developed a gambling addiction, and lost her life savings of about fifty thousand dollars. The noise of the casino allowed her to forget her sorrows. Of course, she was even more confused and unhappy after losing her savings. After seeing me for a couple of years at a discounted rate, she seemed to be doing better. She was able to budget her small income and understand more about the grief that fueled her gambling addiction. Cancer patients need a sense of family to help them survive. If they don't have family, other groups can serve the same function. It is essential that the people and environments that they surround themselves with are wholesome and life affirming.

stopped at a bakery known for its delicious apple pie, and I bought one for Dr. Roeder.

After dropping it off at her office, we went home and had dinner early so that my stomach would be empty for surgery the next morning.

This was my last day with two breasts. Even though I was anxiety ridden, I still made jokes about surgery. I said I was going to draw faces on my breast to show Dr. Roeder how I felt. I was going to write on the left one, "No, no, don't hurt me!" and on the right breast, "You've got the wrong one." I was still thinking that maybe I shouldn't do this. Maybe it's all a mistake.

The Mastectomy

I went for surgery on June 8, 1994, and I was in the hospital for a total of twenty-three hours—a "drive-through" mastectomy. On the morning of surgery, Dr. Roeder came into the operating room and asked, "Are you trying to get me fat?"

I smiled and replied, "A well-fed doctor is a happy doctor, right?" When I had the IV dripping in me I told her that I wanted to put a decal on my left breast that said, "Ouch! Please don't hurt me. Please don't hurt me." Her laughter is the last thing I remember before becoming unconscious. I had a modified radical mastectomy. They removed lymph nodes, the tumor, and muscle. They left one layer of muscle next to my bones. My surgeon did a great job and used very small stitches.

I woke once and saw Peggy sitting in the room, reading a book. I felt for my hat—it was on my head. My throat was dry and scratchy from having a tube inserted in it during the surgery. I ate some chipped ice before dozing off again. The next time I awoke, I had more ice and was asked if I had pain. I didn't, but I couldn't get comfortable either. I was twisting and turning and mumbling a lot. The next thing I knew a nurse was there with Peggy. She attempted to adjust the bed and me, but to no avail. After a while I heard her say, "No pain, huh?" "No pain."

She left the room and returned with a hypodermic needle. "Well," the nurse said, "you act like you have pain, even though you don't feel it. This will help you. I'll just put it into the IV line for you." With that she emptied the syringe into the IV line and smiled. I drifted off to sleep after talking with Peggy for a minute or two.

The next time I woke up, I needed to go to the bathroom, so a nurse came and walked me there. She told me there was a cap in the toilet to catch the urine, and if I needed help to call. I was unsteady, but otherwise okay. Then I drank some 7-Up, which I promptly threw up into one of those hospital-brand, kidney-shaped bowls. I was exhausted and dizzy, so I went back to sleep. I was conscious of blood pressure checks occurring throughout the night but nothing bothered me. Peggy had gone back to my house to feed Vivi and to get some sleep.

By morning, I awoke and was able to eat a little bit and drink water and juice. Dr. Brooks came by to see how I was. Then Dr. Roeder came in and asked, "Do you want to go home?" "No," I answered, "but I guess I have to, right?" "I'm afraid so, but your insurance allows for a visiting nurse to come by once. When do you want her to come?" Feeling very unsure of myself, I thought, every day—twenty-four hours a day, but I decided to behave and answered, "In a couple of days." She smiled, said my surgery had gone well, and that she had stitched the wound very neatly for me. She also told me not to worry about the packing and reminded me to keep ice on it, as I had after the biopsy. She said the nurse would talk to me about the drains before I went home.

It was still early in the morning, so after I was dressed and waiting to go home, an aide came to give me a bath. Well, it was too late. I had packed the soap and supplies because I had already paid for them. I also took my toothbrush, little tube of toothpaste, water pitcher, flexi-straws, and spit pans. At the time I told myself it was because I had paid for these things, but later I wondered if I was taking souvenirs from the fiercest battleground of my life.

The nurse came in and tied my drains on a gauze necklace, so that they hung from my neck, enabling me to walk around with them. The drains are to collect the excess fluid, which would normally be processed by the lymph nodes. They minimize the amount of fluid that is reabsorbed into the body and this allows the wound to heal more rapidly. As this surgery concludes, the surgeon places the drains so that they are in a position to siphon out the excess fluid. Patients usually have to care for their own surgical drains. The nurse showed me how to unstop each one, noting that they were numbered, and gave me some little plastic cups that could hold about one fluid ounce. She also explained that I would have to open up the drains, pour them into a little measuring cup, and record the amount of pinkish liquid released. I would have to do this several times a day and report this information to Dr. Roeder on our next visit. I was also given pain medication to take every four hours for a couple of days.

Self-care can be really frightening and intimidating. How did I know how much of that pinkish liquid was going to be coming out? The amount of fluid is really unpredictable for each individual, but it is always best for it to drain out rather than get absorbed into the system. Each time, I emptied one of my little plastic drain bottles into the cup, recorded the amount, poured it down the drain, rinsed the container, and measured the next one. I had to squeeze the bottle at the end and blow the last bit into the cup. The cups are small, light, and easily toppled, so it helps to have a little coordination The whole process becomes really easy after a few times.

Recovery at Home

Peggy was told to bring the car around to the discharge chute. My wheelchair was rolled down the hallways and out a side door into the hot, June air. The new me left the hospital with one breast, a bunch of bandages on one side, and two drains.

Just like after the biopsy, the most important part of pain management was to place an ice bag on the area. I also took Percocet every four hours for a few days. A pleasant side effect of this medication is that it elevates mood, so I was pretty happy when I was on it.

I had told everybody, "Don't send me flowers because they are going to kick me out of the hospital after one night and I don't want to have to carry them out with me." So instead they sent the flowers to my home. Did they ever! My house was flooded with flowers, balloons, and cards. That meant a lot to me. When I came home high on pain medication, my sense of humor was really crazy. I asked Peggy, "Pile the flowers on top of me and pretend that I am going to my funeral." She frowned, put the flowers and balloons on my bed, and took a picture. Although the explanation for my behavior did not occur to me at that time, I now realize that I was having a funeral for my breast.

After my mastectomy, my therapist and his wife sent a huge flower arrangement. Therapists are usually not supposed to give their clients gifts. This restriction is typically observed because of possible confusion regarding clear professional boundaries. My feelings would not have been hurt had he not sent anything, because he called to check on my condition. But the flowers made me feel like he really cared. Being reminded of how much people cared was critical at this time.

I was also glad to have Peggy take me shopping so I could buy some comfortable clothing. I found some large, loose-fitting shirts that buttoned in the front and obscured my little bottle drains. I also bought a pair of large, cotton pajamas with

Almost everyone is afraid to look at her own mastectomy scar after the surgery. However, I found that the anticipation is far worse than the event. It was not like the movies when a surgery patient has a sudden reckoning with her appearance. Since layers of packing, bandages, and tape must come off before the scar becomes visible, the whole process happens gradually. When everything had been removed except the surgical tape, I could see the stitches underneath. Finally, they were removed after several weeks.

buttons since I could not raise my arm to get into my nightshirts.

The Pathology Report

Five days after surgery I had an appointment with my oncologist, Dr. Brooks. I was high on Percocet, feeling happy that we had everything beaten. Then he reviewed my pathology report and said that all of my lymph nodes had live cancer cells. The chemotherapy had successfully shrunk the tumor before it was removed, but had not killed the breast cancer cells in my lymph nodes. He was certainly more concerned than I was at that moment. There were no guarantees that they had gotten all the cancer. I got really depressed when he recommended that I have a consult with Dr. Taylor at the University Medical Center about an autologous bone marrow transplant (ABMT).

"I don't want to have a bone marrow transplant," I answered. Bone marrow transplants cost money—a hundred thousand or two hundred thousand dollars. They weren't covered by my insurance. When breast cancer patients are exposed to high doses of radiation or chemotherapy, not only are cancer cells destroyed, but bone marrow as well. Bone marrow is the soft, spongy core of the bone that contains stem cells, the immature cells that later develop into white and red blood cells and platelets. White blood cells defend the body against infection and other diseases. Red blood cells carry and exchange oxygen and carbon dioxide from the lungs to the rest of the body. Platelets assist in blood clotting. All of these are vital to recovery.

ABMT is a procedure that removes healthy bone marrow from the patient before treatment and then restores it later. Sometimes bone marrow failure occurs after ABMT. The patient's bone marrow may not return to normal, or may stop functioning after a period of time. Failure occurs if the transplanted stem cells do not reproduce new blood cells. During a bone marrow transplantation (BMT) procedure, a patient's bone marrow is replaced after being destroyed by the chemotherapy and/or radiation therapy. Unlike ABMT, BMT requires a donor.

> If the surgery is a single mastectomy, you may also notices a feeling of imbalance after the wound has healed. It can be very uncomfortable to lie on one side—you may actually tip over. I discovered that a small pillow helped me maintain my balance. As I got better, a king-size pillow seemed to do the job. Size and firmness of the pillow varies with individual preferences. The American Cancer Society and some cancer care treatment facilities provide small after-surgery pillows to help the patient balance and sleep more comfortably.

I was very depressed about the lymph node involvement. I could not think and could hardly navigate the straight, three-mile drive from the Cancer Care Center to my house. I still had to go see Dr. Roeder about getting my drains detached before I flew to Washington, D.C. two days later for an APA conference. I was again disappointed when Dr. Roeder decided not to remove the drains because there was still more than an ounce of fluid draining each day. She said that it was better if there was less than an ounce per day—that there would not be so many complications with fluid retention. So even though I did not want to go on my trip with drains hanging out of me, I did. In the hopes of avoiding the consult with Dr. Taylor, I talked with my surgeon about the existing research on bone marrow transplants. As I puzzled over what to ask him, she said, "Listen carefully to what he has to say, then ask what difference it will make if you have the procedure." I left feeling a bit better. Common sense and straightforward questions and answers are usually the easiest to assimilate at this time.

Eventually I did go for the consult. Before meeting with Dr. Taylor I formulated a list of questions: "Why should I have this procedure?" "Is there a good reason, a special reason?" "If you were me, would you have it?" "How will it help me?" When I met with Dr. Taylor, I heard an explanation of the virtues of autologous bone marrow transplant and put all of my questions to him.

I also talked to several physician friends and colleagues, and did research on the Internet before making my final decision to forego the bone marrow transplant at that time. In fact, since then, scientists have improved the protocol and will continue to do so. Current transplants do not take as long as they used to and they are not as complicated. Now they are often performed on an outpatient basis. At the current time there are some questions as to the effectiveness of these procedures, but I am confident that they will continue to improve. At the time of this writing, the National Breast Cancer Coalition maintains its position that the ABMT's effectiveness for breast cancer patients is not supported by data and the procedure should only occur within a randomized clinical trial.

Friends and Feedback

Exactly one week after surgery I attended the APA Board of Directors meeting. I still had my drains and was heavily medicated. I sat at the board meetings for three days, and everybody said, "Alice, you look great, You're doing so well."

A year later they said, "Alice, you look great. You're doing so well."

And now they say to me, "Gosh, Alice, you really look good."

I ask my friends, "And what did I look like when I was sick? You told me that I looked great then."

They usually answer, "Well, considering . . ."

The truth is, a patient needs to hear encouraging remarks that she has made progress, that she does not appear too ugly or too sick. When giving a patient feedback, tactful honesty is usually appreciated. Cancer doesn't shave off IQ points—she is aware of her appearance.

When It's Positively Okay
to Be Negative

Like so many of my clients, I noticed that during treatment, some people expected me to stay positive all the time. Well, there were times when I didn't want to be positive, when I wanted to shout: "Don't tell me I look great! I feel weak, or lousy, or dizzy, or tired!" Being able to express the full spectrum of emotions during this time is essential. All patients have all too many real issues and situations to feel negative about. It is unrealistic to expect to be steadfastly positive in the face of the greatest crisis of your life. Balance is important. A positive attitude is certainly helpful and should be encouraged, but this does not mean denying negative feelings. It is important to find a way of expressing your anger and sadness without being consumed by them. When those around you can give you time and space to cry or be alone, it can translate into greater autonomy and control over your recovery. This is a good time to begin treatment with a mental health professional.

Removing the Drains

About two weeks after my surgery I had an appointment with Dr. Roeder to have my first drain removed. At the time I was rather obsessive about keeping everything that had ever been in my body. So I told her I wanted my drain.

"You are the first patient to say that to me," Dr. Roeder said. She told me to hold my breath while she pulled it out. It felt like a fire burning through my body, but only lasted a second. Then she said, "Okay, I'll go wash this for you. You go get dressed."

She went to another room where she washed the drain at the sink. When I was dressed, I went to the reception area. With her back facing me, Dr. Roeder was clearly up to something. Then she turned around and showed me a surgical glove on which she had drawn a face. Inside the surgical glove was my drain. She handed it to me and we both laughed. I took the glove and drain to my office and put it on my computer—a bizarre trophy.

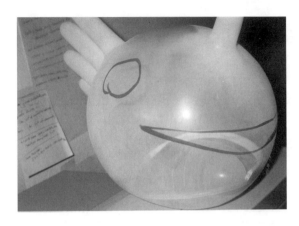

Surgical drain

One reason I share these quirky and funny moments is because fun and lightheartedness can help in the healing process. If you can look at a part of treatment and find something funny in it, even if only in a grotesque or absurd way, it can help to relieve the weight of the situation. While my oncologist was on vacation that summer, I signed up for six weeks of radiation treatments starting in July. I figured that if I signed up immediately and started right away, I could finish treatments the day before I needed to be at the annual APA convention in August. The board of directors met three days prior to the opening of the convention. On the Monday before APA I had my last radiation therapy. I left the next day.

Frozen Shoulder

Six weeks after surgery I was healed and ready for radiation. But first I had to get "mapped" to mark the exact places on my body that the technicians wanted to irradiate. This was when we painfully discovered my "frozen" left shoulder.

After the mastectomy a nurse had given me some self-care literature containing some rough drawings for physical exercises and a note that said, "follow physician's directions." Like many of my clients, I had filed it away to read later. Also like many patients, after getting hurt, I did not want to move. So I did not move my shoulder. Actually, I barely moved my left side. This proved to be an extremely counterproductive course of action—or inaction!

Patients are often instructed, after many kinds of surgeries, to "walk the walls" (see Range-of-Motion Exercises) in the hospital and at home. After breast surgery you have to move your shoulder. It is unwise to let it become lifeless or frozen in place. If it hurts to move it (initially, it will be stiff and painful), and it feels like it can't or won't move, do what you can. Just do a little bit. Do a little bit several times each day. Believe it or not, it gets easier and it will get better. In many cases encouragement is needed, so ask others to encourage you! I have learned to "walk the walls" using the side of my house while standing outside and letting the dog run in her pen.

That July, when I was lying on the table to get mapped, it took twenty minutes to get my arm in position. It was very painful and I spontaneously burst into tears. The radiologist immediately gave me a referral for physical therapy. He also prescribed pain medication and instructed me to take a pill one hour before I came in each day for radiation. Immediately following radiation, I went to physical therapy. Luckily, we were able to loosen my shoulder and avoid further surgery.

Range of Motion Exercises

Walk the Walls

Stand facing the wall with toes one to two feet away from wall baseboard and hands by your side. Place index finger and middle finger lightly on the wall about waist high. "Walk" fingers up the wall as high as you can, gradually stretching the muscles a little more each day. Do this exercise several times each day. Start in the morning and repeat it whenever you get the opportunity. Some women find it easier initially to perform this exercise right after showering when the muscles are warmer and more relaxed.

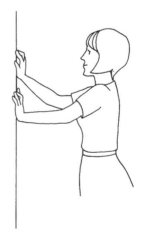

Making Circles

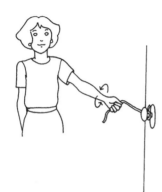

A. Attach a sturdy piece of string or rope to a doorknob and grasp the end of it with one hand. Extend the arm out from the body and hold it as parallel to the floor as possible. Make small circular motions. Alternate circles inward and then outward. Initially, make small circles at about door knob level. Later, raise the arms higher and make circles from the shoulder. Work up to the point where you are doing this for five to ten minutes continuously.

B. Stand with arms out and as parallel to the floor as possible. Make small circular motions from the shoulder. Later, increase the size of the circles.

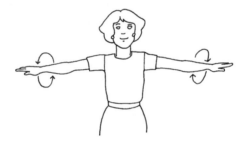

Stick Exercises

Using an old mop or broom handle, or any other long stick, stand up, grasping the stick (knuckles facing out) about one foot away from the body and in front of thighs. Move left and right. Raise stick to chest level, keeping arms straight. Move left and right again.

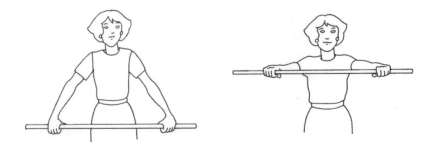

Next, slide hands together toward the center of the stick as you raise it behind your head. Elbows should be bent. Move hands left and right. Finally, holding the stick overhead, slide hands toward the ends of the stick. Move left and right. Lower stick to your thighs to begin again. Begin by doing three to five repetitions, and increase by one to three every two days, until you are doing an average of ten.

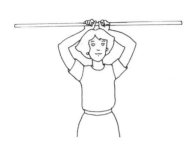 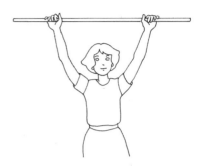

Pulley Exercise

From a medical-supply store or fitness shop, purchase a pulley that can hang overhead and has a wheel that it glides over. Sit under it and grasp either side of the pulley with both hands. Gradually pull one side down as the other side extends up as far as possible. Initially, the mastectomy side will not go up very far, but this will improve over time. Begin by doing a few at time and steadily increase the number of repititions. Do as much as you can.

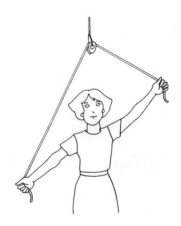

Radiation

Radiation is a special kind of radioactive energy used to detect disease, such as in a chest X-ray or mammogram. It is also used as a treatment measure. In high levels it kills or stops the division of cells. The radiologist will minimize the amount of normal cells affected by mapping out the regions for concentrated rays. Lead molds of the "blocked out" areas are created to shield the normal cell areas and allow the rays to focus on the abnormal cells.

When a patient gets mapped for radiation, the technicians not only tattoo permanent dots on the body, they retrace the lines every day to darken marks that might have rubbed on garments or been washed off during bathing. The first day they take a photograph to make sure they have an accurate record and can check that the molds created for the radiation blocks look exactly like the shapes drawn on the body.

I told the radiation technician that I wanted a photograph also.

I left with my picture and went to work at my office. After working a while, I took the picture out of my pocket and looked at it. I put it back and kept on working. Suddenly I said, "Oh," and turned off the computer. I took my stuff, called my dog, and got into the car. As I headed for home, I said, "I am sick. I have cancer."

From January to June I had not been able to say, "I am sick. I have cancer." Now I cried almost nonstop for a whole day. Like all patients, I had to recognize my illness and grieve over what I had lost. And I needed someone to give me a big hug. About this time in the treatment process many patients

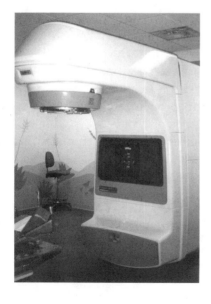

Radiation machine

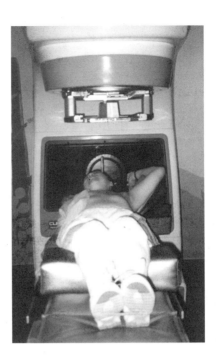

Radiation molds

experience tearful breakthroughs. These are cleansing for the psyche, and a wonderful emotional outlet.

When a patient does not have a family to give her hugs, she needs to ask others whom she trusts. I went to see my therapist and told him, "I need a big hug," and I received a warm hug. I went to see my surgeon. I told her, "I need a big hug." She came out and gave me a big hug. Doctors and therapist still need to be concerned about boundaries, but the boundaries shift with chronically ill patients.

I went every morning at eight to have radiation. After so many treatments, they remapped me. They give different lengths of X-rays for different parts of the body because some parts can tolerate deep rays and others cannot. I was told that the heart and lungs should not be radiated. They carefully tried to avoid creating scar tissue in these areas. But I got a little bit on one lung. It showed up later on an X-ray and neither the radiologist nor I was concerned. It was a small sliver along one edge. I needed to be aware of it so a later X-ray with a new physician would not cause unwarranted concern.

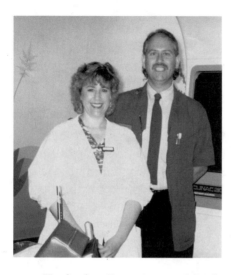

Sue and Jim—my favorite radiology technicians

Each day I put on a thin layer of cortisone cream before putting on the Theracream, which had been recommended by the radiology nurse-clinician, and the radiation still burned me. I did not burn as severely as some patients. Part of the reason is my Asian skin (olive pigmentation) adapts better, but I also took care of my burning. Research shows that darker pigmented skin more readily tolerates burns. It took longer each day to get dressed and undressed than it did to receive the radiation. And I had to go every day.

Theracream is pure lanolin, and I highly recommend the investment. Apply it twice each day and you will limit the burning and pain. Another helpful product is aloe gel. Some of my clients use the purest kind, which is ingestible in the gel form.

For the first two or three weeks of radiation I felt pretty good. By the third week, I was exhausted. Some of the books I read warned me about this. I just let myself be exhausted. It is important to be as generous and understanding with yourself as possible during this time.

Lymphedema

Lymphedema is fluid retention that occurs when there is damage to the lymph system. The symptoms can occur immediately after surgery, after a few months, or as late as twenty years or more after the surgery. It is very important to inform your physician if you notice swelling of the arms, hands, fingers, or chest wall. Some women experience pain and swelling and may suffer additionally from depression due to the effects of their added weight, special clothing, loss of mobility, loss of sexual desire, and worry about possible injury and infection. They may need to wear multilayered compression bandages, practice remedial exercises and skin hygiene, and receive manual lymph massage. With education and care, lymphedema can sometimes be avoided or at least controlled. According to the National Lymphedema Network, anyone is at risk who has had a simple mastectomy, lumpectomy, or modified mastectomy in combination with axillary node dissection and radiation therapy. Not all physicians warn women about lymphedema or appreciate how difficult it can be. In many areas, support groups exist for lymphedema patients.

After the mastectomy and sometimes during or after radiation, patients may experience mild to moderate lymphedema. This can be temporary or permanent. My lymphedema was only a little bothersome and made me forever thankful that my surgeon had the foresight to keep the drains in until maximum fluid had been released, avoiding any residual buildup. I had wanted the drains removed so I could look more attractive, while she had wanted to lessen the possibility of fluid retention. I am glad I listened to her. I occasionally use a compression sleeve, but for the most part I do fine with my extra little pouch along the underside of my arm.

Humor exists even in lymphedema, and my clients love this next story:

> I once had an older patient who had grudgingly gone through a double mastectomy. Afterward in one of our sessions, she said, "The funniest thing is, they removed both of my breasts, and they grew under here," referring to the swelling low under her arms. She was very animated as she first patted her flat chest and then cocked her elbows and raised her arms to show the pouches under her arms, while peals of laughter escaped from her. She had lymphedema and she learned how to handle it, one day at a time.

Introduction to Taxol

After radiation I went to the APA convention and good things happened. My hair was just growing out again. I looked like I had a close buzz cut. I received the APA Presidential Karl F. Heiser award for my advocacy work in the state of Kansas, where I lived while practicing in the greater Kansas City area. It felt good to have my accomplishments acknowledged.

When I returned home, my oncologist was back from vacation. I told him that I had elected to get radiation treatments in his absence because I did not want the autologous bone marrow transplant. He said it was my choice, but he wanted me to be informed about all options. I promised that if I got a recurrence, I would think about it. He told me that the treatment team had decided that to be safe, I needed more chemotherapy. Not hiding my disappointment, I said, "I thought that part of the treatment was over and I was just going to take the Tamoxifen stuff."

"No," he said. "We want you to do that too. But we want you to take some Taxol too. It's a promising new drug, made from the northwestern yew tree. You won't have the side effects you had with the other chemotherapy. You are not going to get nauseated and you won't have lose of appetite and energy. But, you are probably going to lose your hair again."

Because it was so early in the use of Taxol, my treatment team did not warn me that it might cause me to suffer from peripheral neuropathy. No one at this facility knew that Taxol would change my life and become the biggest challenge of my cancer treatment.

Chapter Six

More Chemotherapy: Taxol

Much to my chagrin, I would now start on yet another round of chemotherapy, this time with the much touted Taxol. Before the Taxol treatments were over I would become acquainted with a dizzying array of drugs to treat its effects. I was given Decadron, a steroid used to relieve swelling. To manage pain I took Percocet first, then graduated to Loricet, MS Contin, Nortriptyline, and finally Tegretol. Unlike the experience of 96 percent of the cancer patients treated with Taxol, my treatment proved to be like walking through a minefield.

Catheter Installation

On Thursday, September 8, I would begin my adventure with Taxol, the new wonder drug. Taxol treatment involves a three- to six-hour drip and requires regular blood sampling. Since my arteries were already weakened from all the previous blood drawing and the chemical infusions, I had been given two catheters the previous day. A catheter is used when there is going to be long and/or frequent drips. Certain ones also eliminate the need to "stick" the patient for blood tests.

The first stab did not work, so they had to take the catheter out, make a different hole, and put in another one.

Everything seemed to be fine until I woke up the next morning with my pajamas soaked in blood. Naturally, I was very scared. At six that morning I called the doctor. She told me to put some pressure on it and come into the office. I was able to stop the bleeding. I learned, again, that it is important to feel free to call your physician whenever you need help.

Dr. Roeder asked me if I had received any instructions on catheter care when I went home from ambulatory surgery. When I said I hadn't, she barely concealed her frustration as she called the Cancer Care Center and directed one of the oncology nurses to assist me in this. Later that day I met with Vicki, the nurse Dr. Roeder arranged for me. She entered the room with a needle, syringe, and a bottle of Heparin, along with alcohol wipes and square gauze bandages. Heparin is the substance used to keep blood from clotting. She showed me how to draw the liquid from the bottle, release bubbles from the syringe, clean the end of the catheter tube, insert the needle, and push the Heparin into it with the plunger. It was an easy task. I was a bit afraid of needles and syringes, but determined to do whatever was necessary. To be on the safe side, I would bring my used needles to the Cancer Care Center for proper disposal.

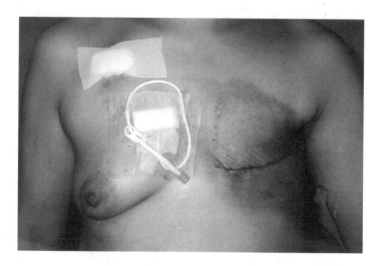

The catheter is installed

Vicki then called the hospital-supply pharmacy and ordered everything I needed for the next five weeks to keep my catheter flow-ready. If you have a Heparin-lock type catheter you must keep fresh Heparin in it daily so the blood does not clot and block the tube. This catheter in my chest was a lifesaver. No more sticks were required. Blood was drawn out, chemicals were dripped in, and I was one happy camper—well, relatively speaking!

A day or so later, I did something very uncharacteristic of me. I canceled a physical therapy appointment. The pain in my shoulder was back with a vengeance, only this time it had traveled to the back of my shoulder. I took a long, hot shower and exercised it for a while. I would ask my radiologist, Dr. Rogoff, about it when I saw him later that day.

At my appointment with him I was given a cute, little white gown. It seemed like my graduation gown—a short one with ties in the front unlike the ugly hospital gowns that they usually supplied.

The doctor came in, sporting a new hairdo, and asked how I was. I questioned him about a variety of aches and pains that I was experiencing, including one in my toe that had been there for a month. He had not planned on examining me and told me that the pain in my toe would have to go a couple of months before he became concerned. I reminded him that it had already hurt for a month.

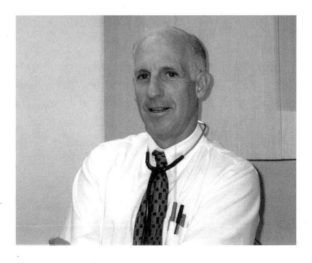

Dr. Rogoff (sans ponytail)

I asked him why my back hurt and he said he didn't know. Then he suddenly asked, "Where?" with renewed interest. I directed him to my shoulder blade area. His touch triggered a wave of pain. When I described the discomfort: he replied "Oh, just a minute. Let's do this right." He did some further examining, asking me to breathe as he touched four different positions on my back to check for pneumonia, which I did not have. He examined my back some more and I felt a burning sensation inside. He asked about the depth of my pain. I said it was mostly just under the surface with some deeper spikes. He then took a look at the peeling skin on the front of my body, and left briefly.

When Dr. Rogoff returned he informed me that the pain I was experiencing was from the radiation and would "go away with time." He also told me to have someone put cream on it. Then he suddenly said, "I really don't need to see you again and I don't want to give you the message that you're sick." The abruptness of our termination surprised me and I quickly accused him of deserting me. He assured me that wasn't the case and that I was welcome to return at any time. He kept patting me on the sore shoulder, having already forgotten that it hurt. I kept trying to move out of his way. It would have been funny if it hadn't hurt so much. My appointment was over and I had completed the radiation part of treatment.

Hello, Taxol

Then I headed upstairs to begin another round of chemotherapy, this time with Taxol. Fifteen minutes later I was having my blood drawn and my blood pressure checked for the second time that day.

It had risen slightly due to the stressful situation. Patients often have slightly elevated blood pressure from the stress of a doctor visit. Then I put on one of the ugly gray gowns and waited for my oncologist, Dr. Brooks.

He began our visit by listening to the four stations of breathing, and commented that I looked good. When I talked to him about my painful toe, he said that he would order X-rays to be sure it wasn't the bone. The steroid, Decadron, that I had started on the day before had helped some but it was still painful to touch. He asked me if I had any questions about the Taxol and I said, "No. I read everything and I understand that I won't get nauseated and that I might get a little muscle cramping, but otherwise I'll be fine." I went to get x-rayed and then reported to the treatment room.

They had gotten some new chairs since I had been there last, including some very inviting recliners. I settled into one of them, turned on my laptop, and went to work. Then I was given Benadryl with Tagamet for swelling and Anzemet for nausea, in a "forced flush." A forced flush is when fluid is put into the vein at rapid speed. After the syringe is put into the vein, the plunger is steadily depressed until it is empty. Afterward the slow drip began. Taxol is a three-hour drip for an outpatient. To minimize swelling, a side effect of Taxol, I was sent home with the Decadron to be taken in descending amounts over four to five days.

The next day I was feeling very pleased with myself. Although I was slightly more hungry and tired than normal, I managed to keep all of my appointments—no small feat for someone who had undergone chemotherapy just the day before.

By evening, which was about thirty-six hours after treatment, things started to change. I began to have more pain. I took some Percocet that had been prescribed for me, but it did not seem to last very long or give me much relief. I noticed that the bottle had a "4" on it, so without looking more closely I assumed that meant I should take it four times each day. After making it through a very restless and painful night, I started taking four per day. The pain felt like I was being stabbed all over my upper torso, and my feet felt like somebody was cutting off my toes and stabbing the soles when I walked. It was the beginning of Taxol-induced peripheral neuropathy.

Nueropathy results when the nerve endings in the toes and fingers become damaged. Initially, numbness and tingling are the most common symptoms. In most cases this is the extent of it and the damage is reversible. For many patients undergoing chemotherapy, this begins in the extremities and moves inward toward the body—thus, peripheral. In advanced cases, as mine would soon become, these relatively minor symptoms give way to pain that can escalate to an excruciating degree.

The effects of the Percocet did not last very long. I drove to Phoenix to attend a meeting in which I had a very difficult time concentrating. When I started to drive home the pain in my chest and arms seemed unbearable. I stopped for lunch and took a pill, and then was able to continue home after about forty-five minutes. I went to bed and slept for a little while before going to a football game with friends. I was in terrible pain by the time I got home and took another Percocet.

The next day was a Sunday, so I only had to wait one more day before I could call the doctor's office. I reread the Percocet bottle and noticed that the prescription was for one tablet every four hours. I immediately tried the new regimen. It worked a little bit better, but the pain still returned before the four-hour cycle ended.

The next morning I dragged myself to a physical therapy appointment at eight. Since it hurt to be touched, I did not let the therapist touch me. I only went to the appointment because I had canceled the one before, and this was supposed to be the final session. Since the Cancer Care Center was between my house and the physical therapy office, I decided to stop on the way home and wait to see someone about the pain.

I arrived at Dr. Brooks' office about fifteen minutes early, sat in a chair, and covered myself with a blanket. An hour and a half later, the nurse discovered me and asked why I was there. I had fallen asleep while doing relaxation exercises.

I told her about the pain, and she said that I was not supposed to have those sensations with Taxol. She called the doctor and he ordered two Percocets every four hours plus a thousand milligrams of Naprosyn per day. Naprosyn is an anti-inflammatory and is successfully used for arthritis swelling and other pains. Later, when I reviewed my medical records, I noticed that this visit was described simply as "unscheduled" and not what I imagined the physician would write: "Alice showed up for a forced visit and complained excessively about unexplainable pain." Again, I learned it was fine to rely on a member of my medical team. I drove to the drug store and got my prescriptions filled. Back home I ate a little and took my pills. I slept for three hours and felt better when I awoke. But my feet still hurt and burned when I walked.

Somehow I made it through the week, sleeping fifteen to twenty hours each day. I went about my chores and got very depressed from the medication. I began once again to realize that this was a real disease, with many medical and practical consequences. I had planned to go to another APA conference and some committee meetings in another week, so I desperately hoped that my condition would improve.

As the days went by my appetite decreased to where I only ate a little when I took my medicine. In the meantime, I tried to go to the office and maintain the household. I was not very motivated, but I forced myself to move around and stretch my tight muscles.

By the following week, I was nauseated all the time. One day I had a meeting from nine until noon. I went to lunch and as I smelled food, I felt very sick. I dashed to the rest room and barely made it before spraying vomit everywhere. After cleaning everything, I continued to be nauseated. Finally, I left and went home. I called the doctor's office and the nurse suggested that I take something for the nausea. Because I would be leaving town for the conference in a few days I told her that I would prefer to see the doctor. She agreed to set up an appointment for me with Dr. Brooks later that afternoon. Everything in my body seemed to be hurting or numb.

When Dr. Brooks saw me he said that he had never had any trouble with Taxol before and that he had asked the drug representative if there had been a change in the formula. They told him there was no change, but I thought the batch might be different. I had heard of someone who did not have any problems on her first round, but was having problems with the second.

The doctor and I talked a long time and I explained that I had a meeting I wanted to attend in Washington, D.C. I did not want to be sick and in pain during the meeting. He changed my medicine from Percocet to Loricet, which he said was formulated with a different base and was not so hard on the stomach. He also prescribed a smaller dosage and just one pill four times per day to accompany the Naprosyn. I left and filled the prescription. I still felt crummy, but that night I slept much better than I had in a while.

By the following day I was feeling much better. Much to my surprise, Dr. Brooks called to see how I was doing. He knew that I wanted to leave shortly. I was feeling better, but not wonderful. We discussed the possibility of quitting the treatment. I really did not want to experience this kind of mind-numbing pain. I had never imagined that pain could create such intense depression. I went through periods of not wanting to live and hoping that I still had the cancer and would die soon. When I was not in pain, I felt like working and writing—I imagined making plans and having a future, perhaps as president of APA.

I left for the APA conference as scheduled but the flight there proved to be an exhausting one. When I finally got checked in to my hotel I immediately took a nap. By the time I had joined friends for dinner, I had taken my medicine and felt much better. Most of my colleagues commented on how well I looked and how successfully I was handling the treatment. Of course I was on Loricet and Naprosyn, so I was able to function. Yet, I often went back to my room for a few minutes of rest that turned into two or three hours of sleep. My whole body hurt and I was having a lot of trouble walking, but I managed.

A few days later I went to dinner with a good friend and colleague, Melba Vasquez, who had a close family member recently diagnosed with breast cancer. I showed her my mastectomy scar, and the "sunburn" caused by the radiation. My back had a big spot on it and hurt a lot more than my chest. I realized that was because I had no one to apply cream to my back, a spot that I could not reach. Melba applied lotion to it and I experienced a lot of relief. I made a mental note to ask the radiation team to be more aware of the help a single woman might need in applying cream to areas she can't reach. I was happy to catch an earlier flight home the next day.

Round Two

October 3, 1994, was the day for my second Taxol treatment. Sitting in the treatment chair, I worked on my computer, sorting messages, writing in my log, and replying to some correspondence. The days following the treatment were rough ones. After about three days, I began to have a lot of pain, even with all of the medication. Then on day four, the stabbing pain and the swollen feet got unbearable, just like the first time. This time I knew enough not to go off to Phoenix for a meeting, or on any other excursions, but to stay close to home. My stomach felt like it was on fire, and I was nauseated, but I tried to take the medicine and sleep.

October 1994 turned out to be the month that I would break my almost impeccable record of keeping appointments. Dr. Brooks and I decided that I would have to cancel my upcoming trip to Asheville, North Carolina, where the APA board of directors was having its fall retreat. I had hoped that I could attend if I stayed in bed during most of the nonmeeting time. But since we did not know exactly what was wrong with me, we decided against it. I canceled my reservations, which made me really grouchy, sad, and depressed. Why couldn't I have responded to Taxol like all the other hundreds of patients?

While I was at home missing the fall retreat, I was not forgotten. During a break in their meetings, I received telephone calls from my friends and colleagues. Many said, "Alice, we realized that you really had to be down if you weren't with us." Other members knew how much I enjoyed the colorful fall leaves of North Carolina, so they collected some for me. Small, thoughtful acts like these were lifesavers.

I had also planned to go to the annual Arizona Psychological Association dinner but could not attend because I felt miserable. I had been having withdrawal symptoms from the lower dosages of Percocet, particularly some very heavy sweating. To top it off I still had some lingering postmenopausal symptoms. It was hard to sort out. From the outside I must have looked pretty silly.

I expended all of my energy just to take a shower. I knew I was not supposed to be this way, but I was more depressed and anxious from Taxol than any other treatment. I often wished that I were dead but would not say it to anyone. No one would have understood. I was in the prime of my career in many ways, though I was not steadily employed. Life seemed so confusing. I was winning awards, getting recognition for what I had accomplished, and yet I was wishing that I were dead. The constant struggle made it seem like living was not worth the effort. Worst of all, I felt helpless to change things. I wanted to help people and to be happy too. I was telling everybody how happy I was, so that if I died they would know that I had lived a happy life. Maybe this would be of comfort to them. Thank goodness I had a psychologist that I could talk to every week.

Another bright spot in my otherwise miserable existence occurred when my friend Christine came to stay with me for a week. She left her husband, Joe, at home in Baltimore so she could rub my feet and run to drugstores buying every nonprescription product that she could find to help them. I still moaned and groaned, but at least I had the comfort of her company. Even though it was not what I believed or taught, I sometimes had a hard time accepting help from others. Also, I had often felt compelled to look presentable and to provide entertainment for visitors. Yet, I greatly appreciated the comforting presence of a close friend.

While I was home feeling sorry for myself, I called my friend and colleague in Kansas City, Dr. Jay Peterson, again. He was familiar with Taxol-induced peripheral neuropathy and told me it sounded like I had a severe case. I asked him about the treatment and he said MS Contin (time-released morphine) was the best that he knew.

Dr. Brooks was willing to try MS-Contin to help alleviate the pain in my feet and legs. My fingers and arms were tingly and numb, but did not hurt.

Three Times and I Am Out . . . Almost

October 27, 1994, was the third treatment with Taxol. After a lot of talk about being admitted to the hospital for a twenty-four-hour infusion, which might have reduced the side effects,

I was back at the Cancer Care Center for the standard procedure. Because the MS Contin seemed to be working, I did not have to go to the hospital. I got to the waiting room on time and then not surprisingly there was a delay. So much of my precious time has been wasted during the treatment process. Then after waiting a while, the routine that had become so familiar was underway.

Four days passed and I became despondent. One of my journal entries read: "My heart hurts where the catheter is and the sweats from the drugs stink, and I hurt from the Taxol . . . and I am not worth saving anyway. I have not had anyone touch me or give me a hug since September 26 at the meetings. It is too difficult."

I wasn't sure whether my ambivalence toward living was due to the side effects from the Taxol, the prolonged treatment regimen, the illnesses itself, or other factors. I felt so unworthy to continue living when I had seen friends with children die. I considered what would happen to my small estate when I died and realized that I wanted to change several items in my will. I wanted to make sure that my niece, Sharon,

The mind/body link for depression works in both directions. Many patients get depressed while in treatment for cancer. According to Ellen McGrath, Ph.D. (1992), mind/body depression is a kind of "healthy" depression since it results from realistic feelings of pain, sadness, and disappointment brought about by trauma, unfair treatment, or past damage. Healthy depression is manageable yet it can develop into unhealthy depression if it is not managed. If you are feeling depression of any kind, consult a mental health professional. McGrath offers some practical coping strategies. Writing about your feelings, or drawing a picture of what you imagine they look like, can be a source of insight and relief. A ten-minute walk can boost your energy and revitalize a flagging spirit. Connected people are mentally and physically healthier, so develop and nurture meaningful relationships. Ironically, helping others in however small a way can give you a lift. Nurture your creativity. This can take many forms and can lead to a richer, more loving relationship with yourself.

would receive some money to help her through medical school. I really did not want to live and I did not know how to tell my colleagues since they kept telling me that I had something to offer my profession and other people in the future. I did not see it. I was frustrated, sad, and, most of all, alone. Loneliness had trailed me like a shadow for years, but after cancer it seemed inescapable.

The side effects from various medications made my life a three-ring circus of complications. Taxol left me with fatigue; joint pain; nausea; swelling; light-headedness; a continuation and worsening of "chemo-brain," or loss of memory; hair loss; and peripheral neuropathy.

Occasionally I corresponded by e-mail with other cancer patients and compared notes. An excerpt from a letter to another cancer patient, regarding the antiemetic drug Torecan, reveals the kinds of mental problems that plagued me: "During my first course of chemotherapy, I had taken Torecan for nausea. It worked pretty well in controlling vomiting. Unfortunately, I set my stove on fire (I live by myself) before I realized how the Torecan affected my mind. I am glad that you have someone else in the house to take care of you—this is a time when it is pretty important . . ." Since I was one of a small percentage of people to have this kind of reaction to Taxol, they were trying all kinds of stuff on me. I had not been able to walk more than a few steps for several months because it was so painful. I missed a few APA meetings because I could not walk, and when I did not have my APA activities, I became depressed. The doctor insisted that I avoid out-of-town meetings until they could pin down what was happening to me.

Most chemotherapy patients experience a degree of peripheral neuropathy and some joint pain. I had pain and numbness in my fingers and all the way from my toes to my knees. The intermittent pain spikes kept me from sleeping, unless I was medicated. When traveling I had to use a wheelchair to make plane connections. I could no longer wear women's dress shoes, which proved to be a blessing. I eventually bought gold-colored, leather tennis shoes for formal occasions and continue to wear them today.

I grappled with whether or not to complete Taxol treatment number four. It is not unusual for patients to vacillate or

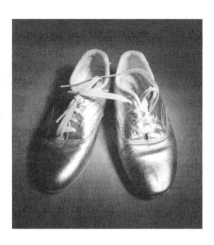

My new dress shoes

feel ambivalent about treatment regimens, especially if they experience negative side effects. We need to be allowed to express our thoughts and be in charge of our treatment. It bolsters the patient's sense of well-being. After much deliberation, I decided to go through with the final Taxol treatment.

The Last Taxol Treatment

Thursday, November 17, seemed filled with disaster as I arrived for treatment. The Cancer Care Center was bustling with patients having or waiting to have chemotherapy. Since Thanksgiving was only one week away, many patients had family with them. Like almost everyone, I wanted to spend my time in one of the reclining chairs, but they were occupied. Only one nurse was in the office that day. I was an hour late for my start time when I finally had my blood drawn. I offered to come back in the afternoon so I would not be rushed. I do not like crowds, especially at a time like this. I rescheduled for later that afternoon and went home. I was nervous and did not want to have the procedure anyway.

At home I wrote e-mails, read correspondence, and took three phone calls from the Cancer Care Center. Each time I received a call from them it was to postpone my appointment for an hour. Finally I received a call asking if I would mind having my appointment first thing on the following morning. In a way, I did mind because it meant that my schedule would be thrown off. I had also spent a lot of time convincing myself to go to the original appointment. On the other hand, I was relieved to have an extra day and did not want my infusion at some ridiculously fast drip. I said, "No problem," because the truth was, it was not a problem for me to drive three miles the next day and I would much prefer to get the infusion at the regular, slow drip, as prescribed.

I took my medicine and slept well that night, reporting for infusion the next morning at nine. Everything progressed smoothly. I nestled into the big reclining chair with my computer and other work at hand, and waited to be hooked up to the Taxol. I hoped that the side effects would not be so bad this time.

Two nurses were helping patients at the center and it was a quieter and less chaotic day than the previous one. I worked on a paper that I was writing.

I hated the idea of spending Thanksgiving alone, but knew that on this treatment schedule I would not be good company. So I declined every invitation. I ordered a turkey at the grocery store complete with cornbread dressing, gravy, rolls, and a pumpkin pie. When people asked me what I was doing, I could say that I had made plans.

By early afternoon I was finished with my infusion and disconnected so I could go home. I had tickets to a dance performance that evening, but my mind became so foggy that I couldn't find the tickets until a week later. I hated for those seats to go to waste.

I filled my prescription for Decadron. This medication has the pleasant side effect of elevating mood and creating a sense of well-being. I thought maybe I would take a few extras since I had the opportunity. Some of my clients used to think the same way, and some abused their medications. After entertaining the fantasy for some time, I decided to take only one extra pill on the first day, and then took the descending dosage, as prescribed. It is not a good idea to arbitrarily change dosages, but for many of us the temptation is still there.

In mid December my MS Contin got raised to three times per day. The pain was unbearable. I was getting very little sleep and felt lousy, overall. Also around this time, Jay and his family drove in from Kansas City for a holiday visit.

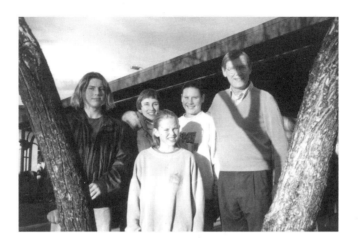

The Petersons

Dr. Brooks suggested that I talk more with my friend about my case. Jay had seen patients with my problem. He understood my symptoms very well. He told me that using the full dosage of Taxol with the three-hour drip protocol created a 1 to 3 percent chance of developing peripheral neuropathy.

"You're Taxol toxic," he stated. He added that the treatment of choice was "to stay off your feet and to take lots of narcotics," until the nerves got regenerated. He suggested that I take more MS Contin at bedtime and a lesser dosage twice per day. I was not pleased with the prospect of a restricted life. However, I realized that if Taxol was this hard on my normal cells, it was probably worse on the micro-cancer cells all over my body and that this might mean that I could be cancer free for the rest of my life. This is a good example of cognitive restructuring, a technique for altering the thought process so that emotions can be controlled. This is empowering throughout life, but especially with chronic illness.

Cognitive Restructuring

What you believe and say to yourself about every aspect of the treatment process affects your mood and health. Certain kinds of beliefs trigger a "giving-up" response. However, this vicious cycle can be interrupted with cognitive restructuring, or learning to view your situation with a different perspective. Anxious and depressed people often think in distorted or unrealistic ways. These distorted thoughts often pop up almost automatically. Learning to recognize common types of automatic thoughts and then to counter them with more accurate and rational self-talk can reduce stress, anxiety, and depression. This in turn can result in less physical and emotional pain, and actually strengthen the body's immune system. Polarizing is an example of distorted thinking. It is an "all-or-nothing" or "either-or" mode of thought. A polarizing thinker might believe that because a tumor hasn't shrunk after the first medical follow-up, it never will. Overgeneralizing is another cognitive distortion. These thoughts usually contain the words "always" or "never." For example, "I'm so sick now, I'll never feel better." Catastrophizing is continually imagining the worst outcome to the exclusion of all others, even if more positive ones are more likely. Awfulizing can be awfully limiting. It is when you exaggerate the effects of a negative situation. Believing that losing your hair means you can't leave the house is an example of this. Personalization can also be a problem. Be careful of interpreting the actions of others as though they are targeted at you. Another destructive thought pattern is tunnel vision. This is when you see only the things that fit your frame of mind and ignore other factors or evidence. If you believe nothing good can happen on a chemo day, you're not likely to recognize the help that friends may have given you throughout that day. Finally, "should" statements are counterproductive. Try to avoid thinking things such as, "I should keep the house clean and prepare meals, no matter how terrible I feel."

Try this exercise in noticing and capturing your automatic thoughts. It is helpful to do this with another person or as a support group activity. For the next two weeks keep a Daily Automatic Thought Worksheet. To help change self-defeating messages, create columns from left to right on a sheet of paper.

Situation	Automatic Thought	Emotion	Rational Response
Cancer diagnosis	I'm ruined	Sadness, anger	Take one day at a time

Loss of Hair	I'm ugly	Self-hatred, shame	Experiment with wigs, hairpieces, and turbans
Friends are trying too hard to show their concern	I have to be good	Fear, shame, joy, anger	It's postively okay to be negative and honest, too
Friends don't call	I'm not good enough	Rejected, unworthy, free	Not everyone is able to handle situation in the way I expect

If you would like to practice this with your family and teach your children to combat pessimistic thought patterns, you may wish to get any number of games and books for promoting communication and self-care. See the Resources section at the end of this book.

I saw Dr. Brooks on December 22 for a follow-up. I told him, "I'm Taxol toxic. This happens in 1 to 3 percent of the cases."

He said, "I'll ask the maker of the drug, Bristol-Myers, about that." He did, and sure enough they confirmed it.

I speculated that my reaction might have something to do with being Asian-American. I commented, "It will be nice when they run the sample on Asian-Americans and find what the dosage level is for them, won't it?"

"Fat chance," he replied. I made a mental note to talk with colleagues about research on toxicity levels among different ethnic groups. Currently, the National Institute of Health has taken an interest in how chemical treatments affect different racial groups.

I started taking Tamoxifen in early January 1995. I had completed my Taxol treatments, but Taxol was not done with me. A year later I was still feeling the pain of neuropathy and taking morphine in the evening. However, it got better after Dr. Roeder suggested the addition of Nortriptyline to my medications in late February of 1996. Nortriptyline is an anti-depressant that has been successfully used at lower dosages for pain management. About a year later I was switched from this to Tegretol for the control of pain associated with nerve damage.

Saying Good-bye

In early January 1995 I went to California to visit my sister-in-law Wai Lin, who had been diagnosed with pancreatic cancer the previous October. She was very tired and fatigued after receiving twenty-five radiation treatments to the pancreas and stomach. She had also had two three-day chemotherapy treatments about four weeks apart. They made her very sick and she vomited a lot. Every day that she was not in too much pain was a good day for her family. She had to rest eighteen to twenty hours a day. Her children had been home for the holidays, which had allowed them to have important discussions with their mother. There was plenty of sadness, yet gratitude for each day.

Wai Lin died on Oct. 1, 1995, while I was attending an APA meeting in Washington, D.C. The night before I got in late from dinner and went to bed. I was exhausted and my "chemo feet" were killing me. I was taking Nortriptyline and MS Contin for the pain and the Nortriptyline kept me wide awake most of the time. I fell into an exhausted sleep at six in the morning. A few minutes later, I sat bolt upright in bed and thought: "I need to call George and Wai-Lin right away." It would have been three in the morning in California, so I decided to wait until later in the day.

It was early evening when I called and my niece Audrey answered the phone. I said, "Hi, how are you?" She broke into tears and she said, "Hi, Aunt Alice. I'm fine, but I'm so sad." I immediately knew that my sister-in-law had died and that was why I had felt the urgency to call. I then spent some time talking and crying with each member of the family. I talked with them about dreams and how they sensed their mother's spirit. Over the next few months they shared a lot of those experiences with me.

George and I talked for a long time. He told me I had an uncanny intuitive sense throughout his wife's illness—it was like Wai Lin and I had our own private line of communication.

He said that she had died at about three in the morning, California time, almost exactly when I awoke in Washington, D.C.

By being able to help Wai Lin's children, it was as though she had given me one last gift. For a while our talks were the only way I could help anyone else. My sister-in-law's death was one of several major losses during my treatment and recovery. Having worked with cancer patients for years, I was aware of the risk involved in being a caregiver or support person. Yet, one cannot appreciate the extraordinary agony of the breast cancer patient as she faces physical symptoms, death of friends and family, and the disappearance of support group members in addition to deaths of patient-acquaintances during treatment. I was able to regain my strength by surrounding myself with positive people and influences as I grieved the losses. I also chose to recognize and affirm the strengths of the people who died. As I continued to improve, I found myself thinking more about the legacies left by each person and I wanted to do more to help promote them. This is a common revelation for recovering patients.

All of us desire that our lives will have made a difference and that someone will continue to tell our stories.

Chapter Seven

Turning Point: My Life after Cancer

Cancer is a hurricane of a disease. In its wake it left my body tired, my mind confused, and my spirit flagging. But like any other disaster it also reawakened my strength, creativity, and will to not only survive, but thrive.

A New Creature

Cancer has changed my body and my life. Memory problems are a common complaint after chemotherapy, but they subside with time. I quit practicing as a clinical psychologist for two years because I did not want to forget the pertinent details of my clients' lives and treatment. Thankfully, I am back at work now. Although most of the peripheral neuropathy symptoms have abated, I continue to experience varying degrees of pain, and this may always be the case. Also, I am told I will be taking Tamoxifen for the rest of my life.

The past few years have been a time for reassessment and re-evaluation of my life. I've had to decide what is really important and what is not worth my time and energy. My patience is shorter. Having been so painfully reminded that time is limited, I am far less willing to squander any of it. It has also changed the way I work with my clients. I was always

Tamoxifen interferes with estrogen activity. It has been used for nearly twenty years to treat advanced breast cancer, and more recently as an additional therapy following treatment for early-stage breast cancer. Tamoxifen helps to prevent or delay recurrence by impeding the binding of estrogen to "estrogen sensitive" breast cancer cells. This stops them from growing and dividing. While Tamoxifen blocks estrogen to breast tissue, it acts like a weak estrogen in other body systems, decreasing the risk of osteoporosis and heart disease. Its most common side effect is hot flashes, such as those experienced with menopause. In some women who are nearing menopause, the drug prompts the onset of it. Other common side effects include irregular periods, vaginal dryness, and weight gain. Additionally, women using Tamoxifen may have a slightly higher risk of developing cataracts. Eye exams at least every two years are recommended. Many experts also believe that there is an increased risk of uterine cancer. However, the consensus among cancer specialists is that the benefits of the drug outweigh the risks. All women taking Tamoxifen should have regular gynecological exams.

rather direct in therapy. Since I have always worked with medical patients, I've had to adopt a therapeutic style that is different from that used in traditional analysis. I am more direct than ever before. If I think a patient will be helped by it, I will also disclose some of my own story, and I do so unapologetically. Of course, there are some personal details that have no place in the consultation room and I keep them out of it. But I don't hesitate to provide an insider's view of illness if I think it can help a client through a tough time.

I have learned to step back and look at the big picture, and to refrain from excoriating myself for every small error or imperfection. As a result of this, I have developed better time-management skills. To my delight, having less inner turmoil has also resulted in a more attractive and youthful appearance. Rather than obsessing about upcoming deadlines and incomplete tasks, I simply let it go. I know it will get done and get done well. In the past, performance anxiety over the simplest presentation or project kept me awake for days. Now I face them with an invigorated sense of self-confidence. If listeners enjoy a presentation I have given, I am thankful. If they haven't, I welcome their feedback. I have truly become more patient with myself, and am more able to practice the self-love that I encourage in my clients.

With cancer I work from day to day. I begin each new day enthusiastic about its possibilities. If something negative develops, I try to figure out how to turn it around and salvage the day. Cognitive reframing has become a powerful coping mechanism for me.

Something Just for Me

To celebrate my fifty-second birthday in 1995, I had my ears pierced at an upscale jewelry shop. Why did I decide to take the plunge at this point in my life? From childhood, I had decided that I never wanted anything in my ears. I had also been taught that it created a cheap appearance. Even then, I did not believe that. But as an adolescent, I had pimples in my ears instead of on my face and I suspected that they would get worse after piercing. I thought my ears were ugly and never had a need to look at them since I had long hair, so I was not going to waste any time on them.

Then I lost my hair twice in one year. The first time no one saw me who cared about how I looked, and Dee and Robert kept telling me how nicely my head was shaped. When my hair began to grow in people complimented me on now nicely my close-cropped hair framed my face. They reminded me that others paid lots of money to have hair like mine. A few times, some people who didn't even know I had cancer complimented me on my hip "mod" cut. I laughed to myself as I thanked them. It was my little secret.

Then one day when my hair was still very short, my friends the Henion's and I had a telepathic moment. We looked up at each other and said, "Pierced ears?" I looked at my ears and imagined small things adorning them. When I mentioned to Dee and Robert that I had tried clip-on earrings in high school Bob anticipated my feelings about them, "You hated it and thought you looked terrible."

"Yes," I said. "How did you know?"

"Because you have very cute ears and don't have enough of a lobe for clip-ons," Dee guessed, and I decided then and there to give myself a birthday gift of pierced ears.

I had to attend APA meetings during my birthday. When I met my friend and colleague Melba I asked, "Do you think I'd look good with pierced ears?"

"Yes, you have nice-looking ears," she answered. A few days went by and on a Friday evening at a little dinner celebration, Melba took out a gold gift-wrapped box and gave it to me. Inside was a pair of fourteen-karat gold studs for my ears. She said that I would need them after I got my ears pierced.

I was really moved and began to feel a little anxious. After all, now I was really committed! The anxiety stayed with me for the rest of the weekend. After the APA conference, I saw my friends Joe and Christine in Baltimore. I showed them the earrings and asked them where I could get my ears done. We went shopping and stopped at a nice jewelry shop that referred us to another one. We went to it, and I proceeded to give myself a lovely birthday gift. First, the woman working there marked my ears and we checked to see that it was in roughly the same spot on each ear. I looked at the little sterile studs as she put them in the gun and before I knew it both ears were pierced. A little sting and burning and then I had two cubic zirconium, gold-filled studs in my ears. We stopped at a drugstore and later Christine showed me how to care for them. I was pleased to turn fifty-two with studs in my ears. I quickly discovered that I had expensive taste in earrings. Most of the ones I liked seemed to be fourteen- or twenty-four karat gold. Taking care of my newly pierced ears reminded me of taking care of the catheter, which I conscientiously cleaned and rotated for six weeks.

Piercing my ears was about doing something daring, fun, and luxurious for myself. It also proved to be analagous to the events of my recent life. The piercing was painful but the outcome was valuable—something good came from my pain. Doing things purely for myself had not been part of my repertoire for a long time.

Speaking Up and Out

As I began to increasingly share my cancer experience with others, a couple of colleagues, Lillian and Fred, began to encourage me to tell my story publicly. Gwen at the APA Women's Programs division encouraged me to present with other professionals, so along with an interdisciplinary panel I gave a presentation entitled "Both Sides of the Bed." I even convinced Dr. Roeder to participate in it. What this presentation drove home the most was the value of speaking out. It was just a beginning. From then on, I talked more, did more, and eventually wrote this book. Presenting in front of small groups that allowed for easy dialogue proved a perfect forum for me.

Spiritual Renewal

Serious illness changes lives. In a breast cancer patient, the changes in outlook are often alarming, especially if she previously fit the Bernie Siegel M.D.(1990) profile of the breast cancer patient: someone who is caring and concerned for others at the expense of her own needs. Comments about these changes may lead to profound and scary questions of identity. Of course, not all women are affected in the same way or to the same degree. While some find their worldviews and personalities barely altered, the change in others may be so radical that it leaves family and friends asking, "Who stole my mom/wife/sister/best friend?" Uncharacteristic anger, shyness, and withdrawal are not uncommon. Nor are changes in personal philosophy. Some women who were always described as adventurous and risk taking may now seem timid and hesitant. The reverse is also possible. This is an opportune time for you and your loved ones to begin therapy.

Many people find that their journey with cancer has brought them to a new place in their spiritual lives. While some are dismayed to find their long-held beliefs shaken, others develop a new appreciation for all that nurtures their spirits. Cancer did not change my belief in or connection to a spiritual power outside of myself. I have always recognized a spiritual power and continue to do so. However, I did wonder why I, a person who strove to be good, got cancer. It is a question that I could not resist asking, but ultimately there is no solid answer for it. My appreciation for music, art, friendship, and laughter has never been stronger. Beauty and intimacy are gifts that strengthen my resolve to live and enhance the passion that I have for my work. I encourage my clients to acknowledge the part that spirituality can play in their healing and recovery, and then develop ways to express their faith.

A spiritual part of my experience occurred during the practice of "healing touch" with my friend Robert. During some of Robert and Dee's visits to my home, we talked at length about healing and Robert invited me to try healing touch. I had also participated in a continuing education workshop in the seventies called "Touch for Healing" and found it fascinating. Healing touch is also known as "laying on of hands." The healer touches or holds his or her hand(s) over you while reciting a prayer or meditating. The communication and trust established through the years of our friendship proved to be affirming and energizing for all of us. Although I have found some of the practices of alternative medicine to be effective in relieving some physical and emotional pain, it is imperative to remember that they are in no way a substitute for conventional treatment. In a recent letter I asked Robert to share some of his intuitive philosophy regarding healing. He wrote the following.

> I understand that this is my reality and others may have a very different opinion. From my perspective most of the work of healing is done by the person being healed. I believe that we become ill because of blocked energy patterns. These patterns may be either physical, mental, metaphysical, or any combination of the three. I have come to believe that all three are spiritual in nature. I think that the blocked energy patterns are rooted in living a life based on "nonserving beliefs." That is, beliefs that no longer suit the fulfillment of one's current needs and desires.
>
> When I have treated you, I have used dowsing to sense where energy blockages have occurred. Then I have used the placement of hands to create a circuit that runs through you and me. I try to focus the

energy flow and keep it going. If all goes well, the blockage gives way and the energy pattern is restored. The person administering this hands-on approach benefits by the flow of energy as much as the one being worked on. It is during these moments of intense healing that we can truly sense our oneness with each other and with the universe.

While the Henions were visiting, before I had surgery and was still experiencing pain, Robert had silently held his hands above my chest in a spiritual exercise. I remember feeling very connected and when we shared our thoughts and feelings afterward, we even had identical imagery. Most importantly, this ritual helped me to feel better. I commented that it would be great if we could figure out a way to approximate this process when they were not with me. That got Robert and Dee thinking. Later they sent me a pair of decorated, rice-filled, cotton glove "hands" that contained pieces of minerals and gems considered to have healing properties.

The right palm contained green tourmaline crystals, which stimulate the physical to utilize greater spirit force. In the index finger was lapis lazuli to encourage the release of old memory patterns and healing of emotional wounds. The middle finger held aquamarine, which enhances the connection to higher self and understanding of universal truth. The ring finger contained quartz crystals to amplify my energy and align it with that of the universe. In the little finger was sugalite, which heightens the sensitivity to the mind/body connection. The thumb held amber to help draw out negative energy and disease from the body. The left hand was another treasure trove of gemstones. In the palm were emeralds to raise appreciation of the unknown and aid understanding of universal laws. The index finger contained fluorite to minimize disorder and stabilize mental, physical, and spiritual systems. Periodot was in the middle finger. It represents the heart chakra. It also furthers understanding of life's changes. The ring finger held amethyst crystals, which lend stability and strength, and promote well-being. Garnet, "the stone of health," was in the thumb. It helps transform negative energy into positive, and reinforces a sense of commitment to self, others, and all positive pursuits.

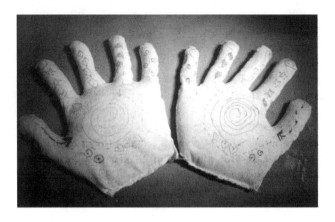

Gloves made by the Henions

Self-permission is an important element. If I did not allow myself to be open or to try, the energy would not flow or remain fluid. This process requires trust, and trust has a fleeting nature. This is energy that cannot be measured, but can be seen, heard, felt, shared, and is usually experienced as a manifestation of love. If we are lucky, we find enduring self-love and, from this, are inspired to help others.

Each individual has a different faith that may or may not have something to do with any traditional, organized religion. The trauma of any illness, especially chronic, unpredictable illness, often prompts us to re-examine our philosophy of life. Whether my clients see this as a beginning, an evolution, or an end of a certain belief system, it is always helpful to take stock of their faith with them. This is a time when clients often reaffirm feelings for love ones. Declarations such as "I love you," "I know that we have hurt each other," "I forgive you and hope that you forgive me," "I think a great power (whether it be Jesus, Allah, Spirit Father, or something entirely particular to the individual) has blessed us with this time together" are not uncommon.

I have found that it is counterproductive to force a spiritual belief system on someone. It is easier for her and her family to formulate their own beliefs. The spiritual healing methods or influences are selected by patients and their families for their own particular and unique reasons. These can include prayer circles by friends and colleagues, medicine lodges, prayers from one's religious leaders, and so on. As representations of my friends' beliefs in spiritual and naturopathic healing, I received many gifts, including a wonderful stuffed rabbit to watch over me and my room, a big bear to hug and talk to when I was sad, a piece of lapis lazuli in raw form, a small amber heart, a piece of jade, T-shirts, and herbs.

From many sources I have come to understand that I have choices. This is the most important thing to realize when you have cancer.

The Academy of Cancer Wellness

In 1995 I received the UCLA Award for Excellence, and I was told that I could talk for two or three minutes when I went to the podium. My friend, Evie, a graphic artist, made a long scroll that I showed before the crowd. I said, "I have a few people to thank," as I unrolled several feet of parchment. Actually I had a lot of people to thank and now I have even more.

It is important to recognize the accomplishments people have made, even when they are very sick. I didn't know how important that was until I got cancer. I had always said that I didn't care if I ever get any awards. I do my work because I believe in it and I do it from the heart. Essentially I still believe that. But getting awards just plain feels good. Upon receiving an APA award, a friend once said that he did not believe in getting awards, but then added, "I don't believe in getting

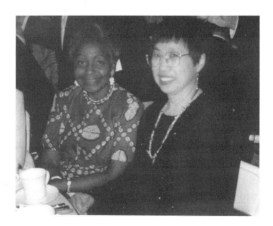

Notice the new earrings.

arthritis either." Accept the good unexpected turns in life, along with the bad.

Well, I got cancer, I received awards, I focused on hope, and my creativity blossomed. The cancer experience has a way of inspiring creativity. When I was sick I decided that there were not enough survivors who knew each other. As I talked to a friend whose wife had recovered from lymphoma, I said, "I wish we had known each other in 1994 and 1995." We both said that there should be a way to connect people. As he described military pins worn for accomplishments, I imagined a popular pin for cancer survivors and their families. This was the beginning of a new nonprofit organization called the Academy for Cancer Wellness. With the donation of a design from a company called Graphic Solutions, and funds from caring people, we now have pins for the cancer "champions" as they complete treatment. We distribute pins to cancer care centers and information is sent to those who request it. We also network on the Internet. The foundation continues to raise money to distribute pins to patients and their families, to create literature for cancer care medical facilities, and to distribute a newsletter. The main research goal is to raise funds for seed money to conduct research on cancer survival.

The Academy of Cancer Wellness issues a credo to all cancer survivors:

You have been challenged with cancer in various forms. Every day you have gained is a triumph. Your success is a living testament to your personal strength, perseverance, and courage.

The foundation outlines its goals in a five-point mission statement.

1. To extend the recognition, among the general population, that many people have met the challenge of cancer and triumphed.

2. To establish a system of symbols that lead to the recognition and celebration of cancer survivors.

3. To provide a means for cancer survivors to rally amongst themselves, for mutual strength and support.

4. To provide funding for research into the extension of cancer wellness.

5. To facilitate the exchange of information, resources, and developments in the field of cancer wellness.

The pins were created in three designs to be given to survivors, family, friends, and/or caregivers:

The champion pin has a blue ribbon, symbolizing the victory of survival. Below it reads Cancer Wellness. In the future, specific colors will refer to specific cancers: pink for breast cancer, red for AIDS-related cancers, etc.

The second pin, a round circle with a rising sun on blue background, is the professional caregiver's pin. This symbolizes hope and a strong foundation from which to serve.

The pin for friends and family is the rising sun, symbol of hope, support, and good wishes for their loved one.

As we acknowledge the accomplishments of survivors and their caregivers, we hope to encourage more healing and creativity. My own renewed creativity has also led me to co-write a play with Paul Donnelly entitled, *Trees Don't Mourn the Autumn.* I am constantly amazed and inspired by the creativity of my cancer clients who express themselves through painting, music, writing, acting, sewing, and sculpting. I have seen an outpouring of creativity from the survivor population. The University of Pennsylvania even has a gallery dedicated to the art of cancer survivors. The potential and possibilities are endless.

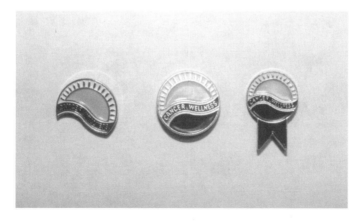

Commemorative pins

Chapter Eight

The Mastectomy Shop

Now I would like to invite you on a shopping trip to some places that provide women with breast forms. I know how anxious and uncertain you may be about what to look for and how to get a good fit for your clothing after a mastectomy.

Reconstruction and Beyond

During breast cancer treatment, a woman is faced with many choices concerning her body. Eventually she must decide if she wants to have reconstructive surgery. For a variety of reasons, I opted against it. In the past, many insurance plans would not cover this procedure, so women were left with little choice. Listening to the experiences of women in a support group or online forum may help in decision making. Some women find that reconstructive surgery restores their self-confidence. Others aren't willing to undergo any further surgery or recovery time.

All choices deserve the respect and acceptance of everyone, including medical caregivers. Insensitive reactions can have a painful impact on a woman struggling with a new body image and tenuous self-esteem.

Unfortunately you can't always depend on medical personnel to be sensitive during this time. I have been told more than one story that illustrates this. The one that sticks in my mind is about a woman who on the morning after her reconstructive surgery was told by the attending nurse, "Sit on the stool in the shower and wash everything to your waist." The patient did as she was ordered. Fortunately, a few minutes later her physician arrived and found her unconscious in the shower. I can only guess that the nurse did not recognize the seriousness of the surgery the patient had just undergone, never mind considering her emotional needs. The surgery is long and quite invasive. A medical staff that is sensitive to this makes it a lot easier.

When and Where to Shop

The best time to go shopping depends on when your swelling and soreness has subsided. I chose a breast form before I had radiation because, having had a single mastectomy, I felt off · balance. I was anxious to look normal, even though I was wearing very loose clothing, and others probably did not notice that I had only one breast. I went to the shop and bought a pair of soft cotton/rayon cups that I could place in an empty brassiere cup. Sometime during radiation I stopped using them because even the cotton was irritating to the radiated surface.

I went to a local store rather than using a mail order or Internet service. The personal attention of a shop is helpful in purchasing the first breast form. However, the advantage of mail order and online services is that you can shop from the comfort of home. This is an important advantage if you are still struggling with fatigue or just feel too self-conscious. Addresses for getting forms and related clothing can be obtained from your local chapter of the American Cancer Society, as well as phone books, cancer centers, support groups, and websites.

I often recommend that psychologists and caregivers visit lingerie departments and stores that sell breast forms. If they're going to make recommendations to their clients, it's important

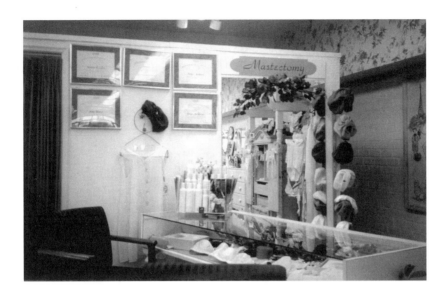

The masectomy section of a local shop

that they know something about the store they're endorsing. I look for clean, private changing rooms, complete with doors or full curtains, and I find out if the staff has been trained in fitting women with mastectomies. Many of the stores I visited had a brassiere or two, but no one trained to make suggestions for a customer's specific needs.

Shopping For "Shoes"

I call this process "shopping for shoes" because breast forms are kept in boxes like those used for shoes. When you locate a store or lingerie department with forms, a saleswoman will first show you to a fitting room and then take your measurements. Then she will bring out boxes of forms for you to try. If you have one breast remaining, like me, then the goal is to match it. If a double mastectomy has been performed then you have a few more options.

One of my older clients who had undergone a double mastectomy taught me a lot about humor associated with selecting forms. Because she was rather large framed, the saleswoman who waited on her assumed that she would want

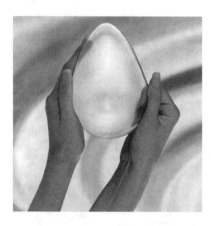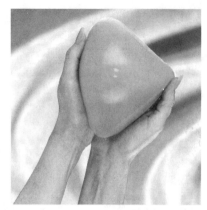

Breast forms

proportionately large breast forms. However, she had always had smaller breasts and wanted to stay that way. She had elected not to have reconstruction because she was older and her husband accepted her current body. Also, she believed it would be easier to detect a recurrence without reconstruction. One day, in her frustration, she laughingly told me that after losing her breasts everything had gone up. I looked at her puzzled, and then she explained.

"When I had my breasts, I bought a fifteen-dollar brassiere or a regular bathing suit. And now I go to the store and I need to get fitted for breasts. They cost from seventy-five to five hundred each! *Each*, not for a pair, but each. I need something altered on a special area for breast form placement and when they sew in the cup, you get charged five each, not a pair, but each."

It was funny and absurd at the same time. Then she talked about how the first forms were too heavy and she proceeded to pull the flexible form from her pocketed bra, showing me her lighter one. We both laughed and said, "This would never happen in a traditional counseling situation."

We had connected, and she was delighted with herself, her jokes, and her newfound freedom.

When I went shopping, the clerk showed me some examples of various forms in my size with a range of price tags. The first ones I tried were too big. We tried several others until I found my preference, which is made by Amoena.

Amoena forms are really soft. If I hug someone, they cannot tell the difference. Also, they quickly warm to body temperature so they are warm in the winter and very warm in the summer. They have a silicone gel interior that feels like flesh to the touch.

After you place a good breast form in a properly fitted bra, then you are ready to consider which clothes you will feel comfortable wearing. In general, you may become aware of closer fitting armholes and slightly higher necklines than in your previous clothing selections. Self-adhesive forms and nipple attachments make it easier to wear clothing that is sheer, and backless, if desired. Breast surgery costs several thousand dollars and maintaining yourself costs quite a bit. Losing a breast is expensive in many regards, but looking balanced and staying active can aid recovery

Breast prostheses are triangular shapes often made out of foam or a silicone gel material in a single or double layer. Foam forms are not the best choice for single-mastectomy women, since they have little weight. Women with double mastectomies can use them but often find that their clothing rides up when they lift their arms. Most silicone gel forms are weighted and sized, and heat up to body temperature. Some forms are constructed as interchangeable for either side, others are side specific. Because lymph nodes are removed under the arm during mastectomy, breast forms often come with a flap that fits under the arm to fill in the space where the lymph nodes were. Forms can be purchased in a variety of skin shades, and with or without a nipple shape. For sheer clothing some women prefer nipple forms that attach with water-soluble adhesive. Some of the latest forms are self-adhering. Breast forms also require care and a special washing solution to keep them clean and must be replaced approximately every two years. They currently range in price from $250 to $500 each.

Well-meaning friends do not always appreciate that a mastectomy makes it a little more difficult to borrow clothing. One very dear friend of mine, who knew that I had breast cancer, wanted to loan me her swimming suit. I felt awkward telling her, "Yours does not have a breast form." However, I was glad to be able to be honest and straightforward. She turned red and replied, "Oh, I am so sorry." I laughed and said, "The simple things are not so easy anymore. Don't be upset." Swimwear requires a different kind of breast form because chlorine will cause the more delicate silicone gel to quickly disintegrate. Swimsuit forms cost about $150 and they fit into a side or top-opening pocket designed in mastectomy suits. These forms are clear, more rigid, and chemical resistant. The swim-suits are constructed with little outward difference from regular ones, except that they have slightly higher armholes and necklines. Some suits come with cap sleeves for those women who have had more extensive surgery. It is reasonable to expect to see mastectomy swimsuits in your favorite clothing stores and catalogs. Many popular companies offer a variety of attractive suits at reasonable prices, plus assistance with fitting questions.

time and build self-confidence. Again, having breast reconstruction surgery is a decision that needs to be made by the patient, not family, friends, or professionals.

Getting Fitted for a Bra

Most women have never been fitted for a bra and don't understand that the first step in choosing a breast form is selecting a properly fitting bra. The information below features fitting tips from Amoena Certified Fitters for their bras and breast forms. By following the easy steps, a woman is on her way to choosing an attractive bra and form.

Items needed: a pencil and paper, a measuring tape, a mirror, and, if possible, a good friend to help.

Step 1. Examining Your Natural Form

Look carefully and objectively at your chest wall in front of the mirror. If you had a unilateral mastectomy, note the shape of your natural breast.

Would you describe the way your breast slopes away from the chest wall on the top portion as shallow? Average?

Is your breast soft with a drape, or firm?

Do you have excess tissue that was left to allow for reconstruction later?

Do you have tissue under your arm on the side with the natural breast that you will need to match with your form?

Write down all of your observations.

Step 2. Determining Band Size

Measure the girth of your body. This is best done with a bra on. Simply measure around the bra band, or, if you are unable to wear a bra, measure the area where the band would be. Make sure this is a good, snug measurement (mastectomy bras must be as snug as is comfortably possible so that the form is held close to the chest wall).

To this measurement add five if the number is odd, or add six if the number is even. For example, if you measure twenty-nine inches, add five to get thirty-four.

If you measure between thirty-three and thirty-five inches, add three instead of five.

If you measure over 36 inches, add only 1 inch.

Write down this measurement as your band size.

Step 3. Determining Cup Size

If you had a unilateral mastectomy, measure from the sternum (the bone in the middle of the front of your chest in between your breasts) over the fullest part of your remaining breast to the center of your back. Again, it is best to measure over your bra.

When you have this measurement, double it. Do not round up or down.

For example, seventeen and a half times two would be thirty-five. Write down this measurement as your cup measurement.

Subtract band size from cup measurement. For example, thirty-five (cup measurement) minus thirty-four (band size) equals one-inch difference.

Step 4. Refer to the list below

If there is a difference of zero inches then you are an AA cup

Difference of one inch is an A cup
Difference of two inches is a B cup
Difference of three inches is a C cup
Difference of four inches is a D cup
Difference of five inches is a DD cup
Difference of six inches is a DDD cup

AMOENA

SIZING CHART

This chart is only a guideline.

Example: If your customer's bra size is 34B:
1. Find "B" for the cup size on the chart.
2. Follow the line horizontally to the square that contains "34".
3. Follow this row vertically down to the breast form style of your choice; the number in this square gives you the size to try.
4. For a perfect fit you might have to choose a larger or smaller size.

	30	32	34	36	38	40	42			
AA	30	32	34	36	38	40	42			
A		30	32	34	36	38	40	42	44	46
B			30	32	34	36	38	40	42	44	46	48
C				32	34	36	38	40	42	44	46	48	50
D					32	34	36	38	40	42	44	46	48
DD						32	34	36	38	40	42	44	46	48

U.S. Bra Sizes®

Name	Style	Side	Breast Shape	Size Range															
Nouvelle	701		Average/Full			1	2	3	4	5	6	7	8	9	10	11	12		
Amoena Affinity	802		Average/Full			1	2	3	4	5	6	7	8	9					
Natural Affinity	845		Shallow/Average			1	2	3	4	5	6	7	8	9	10	11	12		
Delta Affinity	842		Shallow/Average			1	2	3	4	5	6	7	8	9	10	11	12		
Personally	651		Shallow/Average		0	1	2	3	4	5	6	7	8	9	10	11	12		
Delta Personally	641		Shallow/Average			1	2	3	4	5	6	7	8	9	10	11	12		
Luxa Lite	661		Average/Full						4	5	6	7	8	9	10	11	12	13	14
Classic	552		Average/Full		0	1	2	3		5	6	7	8	9	10	11	12	13	14
Classic Light	553		Average/Full						4	5	6	7	8	9	10	11	12		
Contour Tria	444		Shallow/Average			1	2	3	4	5	6	7	8	9	10	11	12		
Contour Teardrop	454		Average/Full		0	1	2	3	4	5	6	7	8	9	10	11	12		
Contour Special	430		Extra Soft Shell	Nine sizes available. Must be fit to individual needs.															

Chapter Nine

Family, Friends, and Flying Solo

When we are feeling healthy and energetic, we're often busy nurturing or taking care of the relationships in our lives. Cancer forces us to slow down and let others care for us. We may not know how to do this, and at the same time fear that no one will. Regardless of your relationship status, coping with people and their reactions to cancer may become as tiring as treatment.

The Best of Intentions

Throughout the whole cancer process, from diagnosis to treatment to recovery, my family and friends made me very aware of their reactions to the illness. There will always be friends and family members who feel awkward and do not want to talk to or visit you. Many reasons are behind these feelings, and usually the least of these is personal dislike.

Like many cancer patients, at first I felt abandoned or shunned because I had this disease. On the other hand, folks who wanted to constantly talk with me drove me nuts because I needed some private time and I was not always in the mood to talk. These ambiguous social situations created many down moments, and yet many happy ones. I began to think about why this was happening, and ways to help myself and others. The reasons why some people are reticent to converse or visit with cancer patients are as individual as the people themselves. The more common ones include a brush with cancer themselves, fears about disturbing the patient, and fears of the unknown. In many cases there is the sense that the relationship is drifting and a friend just disappears. Then there are those significant others who appear at just the right time.

I had a very good friend who I had helped and cared about for years. I thought we had a strong relationship, yet after she heard that I had breast cancer, she never contacted me. To make it more bewildering, whenever this person met mutual friends she told them that she was in contact with me. Initially, this really hurt my feelings and I thought that I had done something to cause it. So I called her and we talked. We had a very positive conversation and she said that she would write or call. However, to this day, I've not heard from her. I occasionally still send her cards because I like her and think that she is a good person. In the past, we had enjoyed doing a lot of things together.

I came to realize that my clients had similar experiences with some of their friends. Friends of patients struggle with a multitude of issues, including feelings of guilt and newly realized fears of death. In the case of this friend, her plate was probably full with chronically ill, elderly parents and concerns about her young children. Since she was single like me, I guess that I had expected her to feel and react the same way that I would. Sometimes as patients, we have to be able to meet our friends and family members on their own terms, or release them to do what they have to. Worrying about these kinds of situations is not helpful for anyone, least of all the patient.

My geographically distant friends presented an array of relationship dilemmas. I wanted to talk to each person and wanted to provide him or her with information. Sometimes I knew the answers to their questions—but sometimes I did not. I felt like I should have the answers, even though it was impossible to know about everything at all times. Friends from Seattle, Washington, to Washington, D.C., said things like, "I know you don't always feel like talking and that you use your answering machine to screen your calls." At first, I had the answering machine in my bedroom, so I would immediately know that someone had called. I felt compelled to answer all of them. As I got more and more tired and irritable, I discovered that my friends were probably right and I should not feel compelled to answer every call right away (an occupational hazard, learned over the years as a psychologist). Sometime during the first six months, I moved the telephone and the fax machine from my bedroom to another room.

One of the most well-intentioned, yet irritating questions I was asked was, "What can I do for you?" I was often too tired to think of any concrete suggestions. Friends and family members often do not seem to have a clue about what the cancer patient needs. Because I am single, I found it encouraging that people were thinking about me.

As I have mentioned, I discovered that I could eat much more easily if I had company at mealtimes. Occasionally it was difficult for me to cook and eat alone, because I was afraid of vomiting. One of the best things that happened during my treatment and recovery was when friends or colleagues invited me for food or brought food to my house. Between them, they provided about three to four meals a week, and there were always leftovers in the refrigerator to nibble on later. With this system, no one was burdened with taking me out all the time and I did not stress any relationships.

In addition, my friend Penny was uncanny about knowing when to whisk me off to the movies. She was careful to take me to the movies that I enjoyed—mostly lighthearted ones. This proved to be a tremendous diversion, as viewing movies at home on a VCR or TV can be isolating. Since my finances were so tight I would not have splurged on this luxury. From these gestures I slowly learned how to accept help from others and conserve my energy for the healing process. Friends who were farther away would phone and send cards, newspaper clippings, humorous books, self-help articles, and novels. I had many former colleagues who sent me a series of books about China, which I loved. They also sent me my favorite cartoons, mail-order fruit, cookies, favorite prepared foods, and teddy bears. I was really spoiled. The mixture of humorous and serious gifts provided a perfect balance. Some of my former clients heard that I was ill and sent me letters, many of which could be summed up as, "Look lady, now you have to practice what you preached." I was really delighted and touched.

Another group of people anonymously sent me money before my disability insurance supplemented my income. Some others offered to help me financially which was really surprising and gratifying. It was especially touching because I did not think anyone knew that I was short on funds for groceries. I tried to save face and reserved my money for medical bills and mortgage payments.

The relationship status of the patient may be ultimately a positive or negative influence, depending on the strength of the link between her and her partner, or, if single, between her and friends.

Common Threads

After researching the reactions of many women, I noticed some strong commonalities.

During that difficult period between diagnosis and treatment, most women struggle with intense mood swings and confusion. The patient may feel especially vulnerable and overwhelmed if she lacks confidants and resource people. With advance planning and by reaching out to trustworthy people, you can facilitate the decision-making process and speed up recovery time.

This period is often referred to as the anxious "limbo period," and is often the best time to learn about the disease and treatment options from as many sources as possible. In addition to getting a second opinion on the diagnosis, referrals from patients, friends, doctors, and cancer centers can help guide selection of the treatment team. Internet listservs and informational websites are helpful. I used both and also called the National Cancer Institute's hotline. For more information on contacting them, see the Resources at the end of this book.

During high-intensity consultations with professionals, it is difficult to remember all of the questions formulated beforehand. This is especially true for the single woman who may lack sufficient support, or the woman who is facing this entirely by herself. I found it useful and important to bring a written list of prepared questions to ask doctors. The company of a trusted friend or relative can be a bonus, along with a tape recorder. I always found it helpful to ask about any tests, especially those that would be conducted on the biopsy specimen, because the results of those tests are used as the basis for treatment. It is also wise to ask for copies of reports and test results, such as the pathology report, mammograms, and radiology reports, to take along for second opinions, or just to have on record. After all, that is what enabled me to write this book. The physicians involved in my treatment had no difficulty giving me my records as I asked for them. Initially, I asked for them in a very suspicious manner because I could not fathom having a diagnosis of cancer and later I asked for them because I wanted a complete record.

All of us must carefully consider how different treatment options will affect the whole of our lives. If a woman is young or childless, the oncologist needs to understand the importance of her future fertility and offer modified courses of chemotherapy, if they exist. (Chemotherapy can cause premature menopause and possibly infertility.) Likewise, lumpectomies are often recommended for early-stage tumors, with survival rates similar to mastectomies. Consulting with the specialists and with other survivors or friends may help you realize your priorities for current treatment and future life goals.

Before treatment actually begins is when you should check with your insurance company and secure all arrangements and authorizations. Some companies require a second opinion. This is also the time to find out about your employer's policy for medical leaves of absence or disability. Then you can delegate responsibilities while you're away from work, and plan a cushion of time for recovery before returning to work. Consulting with other survivors may provide you with a more realistic idea of time needed away from work. Remember, these plans need to be flexible.

All of this preparation may seem annoying and embarrassing. However, the rewards will come later in the form of less anxiety because there is a plan in place to meet your practical needs.

During treatment, caregivers often assume the patient is fine unless they hear otherwise. You need to continue being assertive in requesting explanations, expressing concerns, and describing side effects.

Before surgery, you may want to create a small ritual or ceremony for yourself, either to be done alone, with a spiritual leader, or with a group of supporters. You may feel a greater sense of protection and peace by saying good-bye to your breast(s) and preparing for other body changes. Your hospital room may also feel more safe and comfortable after bringing a favorite photo, piece of art, music CD, or personal journal. Of course, with less than twenty-four-hour stays for mastectomy, you may not even notice the hospital room. For longer hospitalizations, asking in advance about the hospital routine is also a helpful part of preparation.

After surgery a doctor or nurse may show you how to do stretching and reaching exercises to keep your arms flexible. You or a member of your medical team can contact the American Cancer Society's Reach to Recovery program to arrange for a volunteer who will visit and give instructions on exercise and support. A volunteer for single women can be requested. I also recommend that single women invite a friend to stay with them for the first week after surgery. (See chapter 5 for illustrated exercises.)

Three weeks or so after surgery, you may be scheduled to begin chemotherapy or radiation. Some women like to schedule chemotherapy treatments for Fridays so that they won't miss work if they do not feel well the next day. It is important to allow time for rest, since fatigue and depression are common reactions during chemotherapy. And just knowing that there is time to recover can alleviate anxiety. With radiation treatments, which are daily, you need to schedule according to your own needs. Remember, you will get progressively more tired each day, with a low time at the three-week mark. I had my radiation treatments at the beginning of each day, but many prefer to do it later if their hours are flexible or if they are still working.

The whole idea of radiation treatment can seem overwhelming. Some women find it helpful to observe the treatment room and its equipment beforehand. Again, having someone along for the first several treatments can ease some of the fears. Each radiation treatment is not very time consuming, but the entire regimen goes for five days a week for five or six weeks. It usually takes five minutes and whatever time it takes to change from a blouse into a gown and back again. If you do not feel like driving, arrange for reliable transportation. You may want to treat yourself to something special at the end of each week, so you have something to look forward to.

Although every individual's reaction to chemotherapy is different, most women do end up losing their hair. Chemotherapy is another time when you may want to invite someone to come with you, and stay afterward. A hotline counselor and/or a support group may also provide you with support. In my case, the Internet listserv was very helpful.

After surgery and treatment, the idea of resuming dating and sexual relations can seem intimidating. Women often struggle with whether or not a date or partner will find them sexually appealing. If you are single, you may worry about when to tell a potential partner that you have had a mastectomy and whether the news will end the relationship. Some women mourn the loss of their ability to have children due to radiation and chemotherapy. They worry about whether a man will reject them because of this.

It takes time to accept what has happened and to nurture a new sense of self-acceptance and identity. Part of reclaiming your body is understanding that it has been a partner in fighting this disease. Each person is more than the cancer, and more than a breast or pair of breasts. You may require some time to regain a sense of normalcy in daily life before trying to enter into interpersonal relationships again.

Some women feel more like socializing after their hair grows back and they have had reconstructive surgery, or have gotten used to a breast form. They also find that their taste in dating partners has changed. Because most women are selective about with whom and when they share their cancer history, they sometimes find they are more selective about whom they date. You may be more attracted to those that you believe to be mature, sensitive, and compassionate. You may demand to be treated with more respect than before, and probably will want to be more assertive in a relationship.

Developing a personal method of disclosure helps most women to feel more comfortable and confident. Timing and trust are important elements in deciding when to disclose. Some women choose to wait a little longer until they are sure they want to continue the relationship. Writing out and practicing an opening line may prove helpful. A simple, direct statement concerning the diagnosis and surgery is a good place to start, and then add details as the other person shows interest or asks about them.

It is very important that sexually active women who are in chemotherapy use protection in order to preserve the immune system and avoid pregnancy. You should ask for your doctor's recommendation for birth control because in most cases birth control pills are not to be taken during treatment. This is especially true if your estrogen receptors for cancer were positive.

Doctors used to advise women who had experienced breast cancer not to plan on becoming pregnant. However, it is no longer clear that pregnancy increases the risk of recurrence. The chances of recurrence for cancer are thought to be greatest within two years after the initial diagnosis. If you wish to become pregnant later, or to have another child, some doctors recommend that you wait from two to five years after diagnosis.

The Single Woman with Breast Cancer

Certainly all of the aforementioned ideas are true for a single woman. However, a few extra considerations may be more applicable to the woman who does not have a helpful live-in mate. While a single person has learned not to be as dependent on external support systems, it does not mean that they are not needed. In fact, they may be even more necessary for her recovery and health. On the other hand, a single woman is likely to have already struggled with relationships and might have a better support system in place than the person who assumed that her family situation will provide for her needs. Families are usually least prepared for the wife or mother to become incapacitated in any manner, since it is her role to nurture. Sadly, I can remember many times when I have heard from various sources: "If a woman cannot serve and do for her husband and family, what good is she?" This archaic and misogynistic attitude is still alive, even though it is no longer politically correct.

A history of struggling and overcoming obstacles often proves useful for a woman with cancer. She has some fighting skills in place. However, sometimes you're too tired to call up the reserves. At times I needed to be reminded that I was going to be able to cope. A few practical considerations for the single life: being single is a mixed bag. Making decisions about what to do can be a stressor for the single patient who is used to effectively determining her course of action. Having to make urgent decisions about daily practical matters can become irritating and somewhat embarrassing. Such decisions can include choosing when to get groceries, do the laundry, clean the house, make the bed, feed the pets, walk the dog, or paper training the dog so you do not have to be bothered with daily walks. Prioritizing and making decisions about what is most important may be difficult, but it is a process that the single patient must go through daily. During treatment we are often tired, nauseated, and just want to lie down for a nap. One remedy that I found helpful was to buy groceries when I began to feel a little stronger and then cook in the next day or so and for more than one meal. Cooking on good days avoided nausea. Having food in the refrigerator or freezer for those days when I didn't have the strength to prepare a meal was also a big help. The single woman often struggles to apply lotion or cream on hard-to-reach body parts yet she may not feel comfortable having someone view her body. Often she is having difficulty looking at herself, much less having other people look at her. Having trusted friends at times like these is very valuable. Also, the single woman may have no one to commiserate with or to help make light of a situation.

Couples and Breast Cancer

Some women find that their spouse's initial reaction to the discovery of a lump or other symptom is met with: "Oh, it's probably nothing. You're always worrying about every little thing!" He may not be able to understand the significance of such body changes to her. This can abruptly stop communication since he may be viewed as an "unsafe person." Such an impact can be devastating for a woman in this position. She may feel very angry or depressed and wonder, "How would he feel if he developed a lump on his testes? He probably wouldn't be so calm."

However, if she can continue to seek valid medical information, and other sources of emotional support, eventually they may be able to talk more about her physical transformations. Information can alleviate the panic reactions and lessen sensitivity. The spouse's reactions are within a certain context, just as hers are. What would it really mean to him if she had a "serious lump"? Or is it just easier for him to not invest any emotional energy in speculation? It is common for people to catastrophize and initially fear the worst.

The majority of couples that I have seen in therapy have stayed together, grown closer, and placed less emphasis on physicality and more on their relationship. However, women often fear their husbands' judgments. Husbands miss breasts, and it is important to talk about these fears and losses. If the couple can shift the emphasis from this, their future may be more secure.

Often, the woman's fatigue and depression from chemotherapy is a greater detriment to resuming sexual activity than any beliefs regarding her body. Certainly her grief may be causing her partner more distress than any changes in her anatomy.

Usually with some time and work, couples are able to look at themselves and express their affections in different ways. Some of them realize that a body part is not the number one priority. The relationship and communication is. In some situations, the men become vulnerable and stray. They might have affairs, or they may just find someone with whom to share thoughts and ideas. They may leave and get divorced. Some women get divorced because they think they are too unworthy to be married. Diversity of reactions between people who have cancer and their partners calls for improved communication about feelings and thoughts and should include discussion about the missing breast(s).

Spouses and partners may also struggle with their own increased hypersensitivity or worry about physical symptoms and mortality. This can be especially difficult for same-sex female partners who may suddenly realize their own vulnerability to breast cancer. Partners may also feel burdened with the responsibility to be the "strong one."

Talking to Children

All mothers with breast cancer wonder about how much to tell their children and how their cancer will affect their children. Everything that I have described during the treatment process will happen to mothers who have breast cancer. Children will see their mother's nails turn purple and hair fall out. I have seen children who were very scared to watch their mother lose her hair because they weren't told about the cancer—just that their mother was very sick. Generally, the children will acclimate to the comfort level of the parents and other people who are involved with their mother's treatment process.

Crying with family members, and sharing other emotional highs and lows, can be cleansing and healing. As older children begin to help with the chores and with younger siblings, it is important to remember that the teenager is not the primary caregiver. She/he needs to be allowed and encouraged to continue with normal activities whenever possible.

Family meetings and negotiations provide opportunities for rotating responsibilities, or determining what each member is most capable of doing. A lot of decisions will depend upon the family's financial status, as well as the ages of the children and accessibility to friends and external support systems. Spreading the responsibility and opportunity among the family members is helpful for family bonding and cohesiveness. Many children are eager to pitch in and will do almost anything to keep their mother healthy. There is a fine line between inducing guilt with regards to the mother's breast cancer and getting needed assistance.

Sometimes when children feel very threatened or vulnerable they do not want to be near other family members. They may feel helpless or that they should be more powerful, causing them to behave in unexpected ways. A trusted person such as a religious leader, a family psychologist, or a counselor who specializes in working with illness within the family can be very helpful at this time. Close friends or parents of school-age children often can be helpful by just being present for the younger ones.

Daughters of mothers with breast cancer often face some similar issues, such as the fear of getting breast cancer, the fear of losing their mother, the fear of people being afraid of them since they might get breast cancer one day, and discomfort with their sexuality. Group therapy with other daughters of surviving women is one way that girls can learn to cope with cancer.

Family rituals can help ease anxiety and provide comfort for children. Some families use daily prayers, weekly viewing of comedy videos, writing love letters, making favorite meals, doing art projects, or gardening to lend some structure to life. Families can learn to develop a sense of humor about hair loss by having fun with scarves, turbans, and funny hairpieces. Changing the meaning of events attached to surgery and treatment from negatives into positives (reframing) works well for children.

My friend Melba's sister, Norma, was in her thirties when she had breast cancer. Her four children ranged in age from four to fifteen. Since they lived in a rural area, their mother was housed in an extended-care facility near the hospital for several days when she went to have chemotherapy treatments. She always invited any of the children who wanted to accompany her to go along. Each of the children asked their questions at a level that was understandable to them, either individually or among themselves. When side effects of chemotherapy occurred, such as hair loss or the changing color of the fingernails, the children were always invited to ask questions and share. At a glance, this might seem too intense, but it turns out that her children liked to do this.

When it came time for Norma's hair to fall out, she tested it and said, "I'm going into the bathroom to take my hair out. Who wants to come with me?" Eventually all the kids went with her, even though the littlest one was reluctant. They decided to save their mother's hair. They spent about a half hour together, laughing and joking as they removed their mother's hair. Suddenly their mother appeared thin, pale, bald, and very sick. Then the youngest one started to cry. They all cried together and realized how much they needed one another. Soon it turned into a celebration because the mother helped them understand that her baldness meant that the chemo-therapy was working.

The following activities can be used to encourage communication, creativity, and humor. Some of these activities may need to be preceded by discussion about their value and relevance to the family's current situation:

Family Interviews: let the kids use a video camera and ask questions to grandparents and parents about their childhood memories. They can pretend they are reporters for the "Smith Family Network."

Family Cancer Scrapbooks: either together or individually, members can create a book complete with photos, recording the story of Mom's cancer. Encourage decorations, letters, photos, and especially those events that Mom might have missed attending because she was in treatment.

Personal Story of Cancer: the patient or older family members may find it therapeutic to write their own account of cancer and how it has affected her/his life. This does not have to be shared with anyone, although it may be useful in personal counseling.

Mom's "Life Story" Book: these are available at many book and gift stores. If Mom does not feel like writing, a page per day could be completed by a child acting as the scribe.

The "Orpheus Exercise": this original activity was developed and named by existential psychologist James Bugenthal (Spiegel 1993). It was designed to help people imagine giving up aspects of themselves and examining what remained. A variation of it is often used to help people experience the loss of an aspect of life.

Certainly, adolescents, teenagers, parents, and grandparents or support group members could share this together.

1. Write down six or more defining aspects of your life and number them by priority. (Playing the guitar, talking to my friends, going to work, reading books.)

2. Cross off or crumple up the lowest priority item. Imagine that you could no longer fulfill that role.

3. Imagine another role being stripped away, then another, and so on, until you are left with only one.

4. Try to answer the questions: Who would you be if you were not what you are now? Do you have value as a person outside of your career, or family role?

Illness across the Generations

As women share their symptoms and diagnoses with other family members, they may discover genetic predispositions. An aunt may remember a grandparent's fight with cancer, or a cousin may disclose her recent diagnosis. All of this can ease feelings of isolation within the family, but the reactions of the people may be disappointing or non-supportive. Even a confirmation of genetic predisposition can be frightening.

From parent to child, the guilt and anger about inherited predispositions can make dealing with day-to-day illnesses more stressful. Occasionally parents start ruminating about their children's behavior and symptoms and wonder if they are developing an inherited physical or emotional challenge. Helplessness for both generations can start to destroy the impact of positive messages that the children hear. In moments of despair parents are loathe to admit that sometimes they think, "I wasn't meant to have children—I shouldn't have, and now look what might happen to them." On the other hand, children may carry a dark cloud of concern that they are walking "time bombs." Renewed efforts at modeling healthy self-care may be the best approach for known predispositions.

Adolescent girls tend to be especially worried about the genetic impact of breast cancer. The National Breast Cancer Alliance has a videotape that they distribute free of charge to various organizations. While those affected are a very small percentage, the media has heightened the awareness of the availability of tests. Unfortunately, they have not spoken so much about the long-term effects in the current or future job market, confidentiality, or effects on the patient's or family members insurability. Other information can be accessed from the N.I.H.—National Human Genome Research Institute, the National Cancer Institute, the American Psychological Association, and the National Society of Genetic Counselors (see the Resource section at the back of this book).

Family members can also develop angry or impatient defenses when facing an undiagnosed, let alone diagnosed, condition in a loved one. They can grow discouraged while trying to encourage a loved one into better health and habits. Some also become very irritated at the lack of responsiveness. The inability to "solve it" as a family is often the source of frustration and sometimes causes withdrawal on the part of the loved one. Of course this only adds to her feelings of rejection, isolation, and sense of being "damaged."

So, the actual diagnosis is a mixed bag. On one hand their is relief at having a recognized label for the pain and problems that have been plaguing patient and family. On the other hand is the possibility of a death sentence for future hope. Everyone in the family system loses something if all of the interactions become focused on illness, medicine, and doctors—hence the need for humor. There may also be the temptation for family members to protect and not challenge the diagnosed patient, to leave her alone since she might not be able to tolerate noise and activity . . . in effect, to write her off as already a "goner."

An increasingly incapacitated spouse or parent may raise the ire of caretaking family members who recall all those foolish things that the patient did in years gone by that may have added to her present illness. And there is always a truckload of guilt and anger for opportunities not taken (the cruise we never got to have), or a change in the script for the end of one's marriage and life. So much grief exists just below the surface. It sometimes breaks forth in unexplained tearfulness, new addictions, and personality disturbances.

Ultimately, the patient's own attitude regarding her diagnosis and future goes a long way toward setting the climate for family and friends. She needs to learn those important boundaries of time and space that allow her to ask for quiet and rest. On the other hand, clear communication about her inclusion in family traditions and events helps everyone to keep her informed and involved.

I have experienced what I refer to as the "law of diminishing returns" with regards to depending on biological family members for emotional and physical support. As a patient proceeds through stages of treatment, family members may believe that the patient is finally "over the hump" and is getting better. Unless they have experienced cancer, it is hard for them to sustain time and energy for such a lengthy process. The special attention, gifts, and phone calls dwindle while the patient is still fighting for her life. And the family members move on to other crises, cares, and challenges.

I have always believed that a wise patient and a wise person is careful to select a "Family of Choice" wherever he/she goes. This family is selected rather than inherited, and can provide those character qualities that one finds most necessary for living a positive lifestyle. Such friends never replace the family of origin; however, they seem to exponentially increase the patient's support.

Chapter Ten

Understanding and Coping with Chronic Illness: A Lifetime of Experiences

I am one of 186,000 women who get breast cancer each year in the United States. I believe that I have survived cancer treatment, but not cancer. Like many of my clients, I received lots of flowers, cards, and visits during treatment. And everyone had a diet for me to try, a book to live by, or some article I had to read. I loved the shower of attention, while at the same time I felt humbled and embarrassed. However, after treatment there is an unexpected void of attention. Although there is often little support, we still have to consider health issues and the practical difficulties that go along with them.

What's Around the Corner?

Patients worry endlessly about the return of cancer. How do you know which physical twinges to worry about and which to ignore? When my clients who have had cancer complain of aches and pains, I inquire rather directly, "Are you afraid you might have cancer again?" It is important to acknowledge their anxiety because it can quickly mount and become unhealthy. I usually encourage patients to have their oncologist run whatever test or exam is needed, so that the excessive worry does not interfere with recovery.

If a breast cancer patient is going to have another bout with cancer, it is usually breast cancer, rather than another kind, that appears. That does not necessarily mean cancer in the breast. Abnormal cells that are often identified as breast cancer cells can reoccur in the brain, or in the soft tissue organs of the body—lungs, heart, liver, and in the bones.

Other, independent cancers such as sarcomas of the uterus are also sometimes seen. But 90 percent of the time, it is the breast cancer which shows itself again. Hence, the reason for chemotherapy first, if you have inflammatory breast cancer. The first time is the best chance they have to catch it at the cellular level.

The Nature of Chronic Illness

Chronic diseases are broadly defined as illnesses that are prolonged, do not resolve spontaneously, and are rarely cured completely. In most of these, when the patient is doing well, he or she is in remission. I consider cancer a chronic illness.

Chronic illness can generate additional illnesses or impairments. Comorbidity (more than one illness) is most frequent among the elderly because of multiple medical complications associated with aging. Cancer patients often experience a lowered immune system for some time after treatment, and for many this is a permanent condition. This results in a greater risk of infection. A common complaint from my clients who have had mastectomies is that they get many more infections than in the past. Also they are more susceptible to the common cold and viruses, and in some cases extreme swelling can be debilitating. In addition, when they sustain a small cut (like a paper cut, or a nick) the opening does not heal readily, but rather festers and swells. In the past, they just rinsed off the superficial wound with water and maybe applied an adhesive bandage, but now they must be sure to use some antibacterial ointment. Although these are usually just nuisances, this sort of irritation can become a source of stress and increase your sense of vulnerability.

Lymphedema is another chronic problem. The patient's response depends on the severity of her case, time of detection, hygiene, and the availability of lymphedemic massage. In some cases the swelling can be debilitating and in others it's merely annoying. Swollen limbs often lead to swelling in other parts of the body.

> Early in my professional life, I had a patient who complained of leg, stomach, and arm swelling, which was very painful. In my naivete, I blithely suggested, "Just elevate it and it will go down." This chronic condition was relieved by elevation, but a more effective solution was suggested by a physical therapist. She recommended massage to help the fluids circulate until they could leave the body. This provided tremendous relief. However, when a lifelong treatment regimen was recommended, she became depressed and had difficulty coping. We spent some time incorporating the massages into her life and after she had adjusted her schedule, her outlook improved. She could see the "temporary light at the end of the tunnel." Over time, when regular massages were integrated into her schedule, she did not have to be in unbearable pain before her condition was treated.

Depression, even debilitating depression, often accompanies chronic illnesses, especially when the patient ruminates on the likelihood of never being "cured." These illnesses challenge families, patients, and the medical and psychological professions on many levels.

Six Basic Ways to Cope

Psychologists and other mental health care providers have an enormous role in helping patients, their families, and their employers understand and provide the necessary support to promote wellness and productivity. Over the last twenty years I have worked with cancer patients and others with chronic illnesses such as heart disease, pain management, severe asthma, emphysema, renal failure, and chronic fatigue syndrome. I have learned a lot about providing relief for people with chronic maladies. I believe that there are six basic ways to cope with living after treatment.

1. **Understand who is providing the follow-up care.** Ideally, follow-up should be handled by the doctor that you like best, and then she or he will communicate with the other physicians and providers on your team. However, this may not always be possible given the current health care system. You can expect to have X-rays once a year after cancer, and mammograms twice yearly for the first two years, then less frequently. It is unwise to put off mammograms if you have had cancer. If you are taking Tamoxifen to inhibit estrogen production, it is usually recommended for five years. I will have to take it for the rest of my life because of the severity of my specific disease. Tamoxifen helps build bone and prevents heart disease. I found out that I have osteoporosis (not uncommon in Asians because we tend to have smaller bones and less bone mass from the beginning). Tamoxifen and Fosamax have helped me to regain at least 2 percent of my bone mass. This was assessed via a dex bone density scan.

   A concern for breast cancer survivors taking Tamoxifen is the possible increase in susceptibility to uterine and ovarian cancer and Alzheimer's disease. It becomes even more imperative to get regular pap exams, even though you may not feel like doing so. Get regular pap smears regardless of your age or sexual involvement. I was attending a conference when I heard about the possibility of Tamoxifen making a patient more vulnerable to Alzheimer's disease. I over-

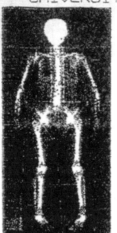

UNIVERSITY MEDICAL CENTER

May 3 09:24 1995 [333 x 152]
Hologic QDR-2000 (S/N 2392)
Enhanced Array Whole Body V5.68A

	D85839S0A	Wed May 3 09:13 1995
Name:		ACHA
Comment:		
I.D.:	2912157C	Sex: F
S.S.#:	- -	Ethnic:
ZIP Code:		Height:5' 3"
Scan Code:	115	Weight: 134
BirthDate:	82/17/43	Age: 52
Physician:		WHI

Image not for diagnostic use

TOTAL BMC and BMD CV is < 1.8%
C.F.   1.018   1.001   1.000

Region	Area (cm2)	BMC (grams)	BMD (grams/cm2)
L Arm	182.35	122.37	0.671
R Arm	185.16	132.86	0.718
L Ribs	38.73	44.27	0.548
R Ribs	89.57	53.36	5.596
T Spine	179.14	135.24	0.755
L Spine	53.02	45.85	0.858
Pelvis	163.88	161.14	0.983
L Leg	349.04	355.27	1.015
R Leg	346.63	362.15	1.045
SubTot	1638.33	1411.71	0.866
Head	259.47	532.76	2.053
TOTAL	1889.88	1944.47	1.829

HOLOGIC

UNIVERSITY MEDICAL CENTER

Hologic QDR-2000 (S/N 2392)
Enhanced Array Whole Body V5.68A
May 3 09:24 1995

	D85839S0A	Wed May 3 09:13 1995
Name:		ACHA
Comment:		
I.D.:	2912157C	Sex: F
S.S.#:	- -	Ethnic:
ZIP Code:		Height:5' 3"
Scan Code:	115	Weight: 134
BirthDate:	82/17/43	Age: 52
Physician:		WHI

T0AR581
F.S. 68.00% 0(10.00)%

Region	BMC (grams)	Fat (grams)	Lean (grams)	Lean+BMC (grams)	Total (grams)	% Fat (%)
L Arm	122.4	1485.1	1731.1	1853.5	3338.6	44.5
R Arm	132.9	1218.8	1701.7	1834.6	3045.3	39.8
Trunk	439.1	8227.4	28377.2	28816.3	29043.7	28.3
L Leg	355.9	3882.4	6144.8	6500.8	10382.2	37.4
R Leg	362.2	3954.3	6173.9	6536.1	10498.4	37.7
SubTot	1411.7	18759.7	36128.7	37540.4	56300.2	33.3
Head	532.8	838.8	3250.8	3783.6	4621.6	18.1
TOTAL	1944.5	19597.7	39379.5	41324.0	60921.8	32.2

*assumes 17.8% brain fat
LBM 73.2% water

HOLOGIC

Bone density scan

heard some women without breast cancer or a history of breast cancer flippantly say that they would never take Tamoxifen and would rather have breast cancer than Alzheimer's. That was interesting to those of us who had been through treatment, or who had a loved one with a history of breast cancer. Those of us in this position often respond to those comments by saying, "Alzheimer's usually runs in families and I would check family history before making the decision." Having gone through the treatment, it seemed easier to want to avoid a recurrence of the breast cancer. These bits of news keep a patient hypervigilant and can add to the stress of the illness and everyday living.

2. **For every action there is a reaction.** Patients do have some control. The media seems to be a constant threat to some of my clients and to many survivors. Evening after evening they allow their minds to be bathed in the negative wash of the news. They may get tense, anxious, or sad. They may read something about breast cancer and get upset because the discovery was not available during their treatment, or they may question why so many people are still suffering. The good news is that there is a course of action. If you are troubled by what you're reading or watching, put down the article, change the channel, or turn off the television. You can learn to pay attention to your own signals that something is upsetting—the tense muscles, agitation, or despair. We really can choose as we consider the consequence of each behavior.

3. **Keep on plodding.** The importance of this maxim was made clear to me as I worked with clients over the years. My brother was the first to phrase it this way to me. He and I e-mailed encouragement to each other over a two-year period. "Keep on plodding" became like a mantra, which encouraged us to go forward and continue to try even when we felt tired, sad, or desperate.

4. **Get empowered to make decisions.** Getting empowered to make decisions comes from many different

sources. It may be as simple as repeating "Keep on plodding" to yourself, or it may come from effecting a change in direction, attitude, or environment. Get the information and support you need to be empowered.

5. **Discover the value of humor.** Laughter really is the best medicine. Family and friends also need humor. Remember that there are individual differences in how it is expressed. While using intuition and sensitivity, therapists and others can often employ humor to move the focus of the conversation. Patients often forget that they are able to transform their emotions, and humor tends to facilitate great breakthroughs.

6. **Ask for your space.** Family members need to know that it is okay for the patient to want to be alone, and that it does not mean that she is necessarily depressed. You may want solitude to think, read, meditate, watch a movie, listen to music, rest from conversation, laugh, cry, or pray. You have every right to ask for and be granted this time. A patient does not lose the opportunity to choose because she is ill. I encourage independence and dignity in living whenever possible.

Chronic Illness and Health Care Providers

Just like everything else in life, my perceptions of the medical system have changed since getting cancer. I am fairly certain that I received deferential treatment from my health care providers. I did not have as many obstacles because I spoke out and asked questions. Also, as a psychologist who works with medically ill patients, I was

As an Asian-American woman with breast cancer, I experienced a double whammy. While I was undergoing the trauma of treatment, many people expected me to be subordinate, inscrutable, and unfailingly stoic. So often my opinions were discounted, and when I got angry about it I was "making a big deal out of a nothing." My experience is not unlike that of many of my female clients and those of underrepresented groups, whether or not they have breast cancer.

more knowledgeable from day one. I informed everyone that I was very active in health care reform, and that I was going to Washington several times in an attempt to effect change in our health care system. Physicians are like most of us—they tend to be more helpful if we ask questions and let them know our needs. In my case, I needed them to know that I intended to make a difference in health care in both the local and national arenas. Also, I needed a little flexibility in my treatment schedule because it was important for me to remain active.

Doctors can seem larger than life. Many patients feel indebted to their surgeon or physician and do not want to "bother" him or her. If funds and resources are limited, treatment choices can be even more difficult. Individuals vary in their comfort level about how to approach doctors. There is not one set prescription for how to talk to them. However, most appreciate questions and hearing what their patients have to say, even though their time may be limited.

Fortunately, I did not have any doctors who became angry because I asked questions, as I worried they might. Some will get impatient or angry for any number of reasons. If the doctor is a skillful surgeon or a good technician and you want to be treated by him or her, find a way to be comfortable with his or her personality. In addition, find someone else to talk to. A therapist or counselor is often more prepared to talk about how to approach people. I really questioned my doctors a lot and I feel good that I was able to do that, even though from time to time I scared myself with my newfound assertiveness.

The High Price of Chronic Illness

Chronic health concerns have been of primary interest in the United States since the early 1920s because they affect the workforce and usually prove to be life threatening at some point. These chronic health concerns include both diseases and impairments. In addition to the physical aspect, there has always been the financial concern. The cost of caring for the chronically ill continues to escalate, especially in an age when longevity is flourishing. Thus, quality of life and productivity become major concerns. Psychological well-being has played a huge role in the lives of my clients and their families.

We all want to live with dignity. Sometimes people with chronic conditions can continue their careers and jobs. The managers concerned about "bottom line" issues tend to approach such employees from a different perspective than the psychosocial folks do. The flextime positions that have been urged for working mothers would probably benefit chronically ill patients as well. The end result would probably be a viable, functioning population that does not present an overwhelming burden to the family, the employer, or the health care system.

The Chronic Illness Equation

Coping with chronic illness reminds me of the Chinese character for "crisis." The character is actually composed of two words: "danger" and "opportunity." Most of my patients describe coping with chronic illness as including an element of danger. As we examine and reevaluate this, we often find areas of opportunity that can add a positive perspective to coping. This may not be so apparent from the outset, but by using cognitive restructuring, you can successfully cope. If you are not accustomed to looking at things from a positive perspective, you need to be vigilant and take advantage of opportunities. By adopting this attitude of crisis = danger + opportunity, we can encourage our friends, relatives, and others to accompany us, rather than control us in our journey.

Chapter Eleven

Questions and Answers

As I crisscross the country giving lectures and seminars about breast cancer, I am asked a multitude of questions by professionals and cancer survivors. Below are some of the most common ones.

Q: Do you currently experience any side effects from treatment?

A: I am not experiencing many side effects other than some remaining Taxol-induced peripheral neuropathy, especially in my feet. One other side effect that has become a way of life for me is the night sweats. While they're not nearly as bad as they were at the beginning of chemotherapy, I am usually awakened once a night by them. I know that at about two-thirty or three in the morning I will wake up in a sweat. However, considering the alternatives, this is not such a big deal. I have learned to live with it.

Q: How long does one take Tamoxifen?

A: Initially, it was believed that Tamoxifen should be taken for one to five years. Now, if you have had inflammatory breast cancer and/or a history of breast cancer, the recommendation is for indefinite treatment with Tamoxifen. I am not aware of any research concerning diminished returns.

Q: Does chemotherapy affect a woman's hormones?

A: Yes. Chemotherapy and the trauma of treatment in general can result in the patient having reactions similar to that of a menopausal woman. Because hormone production has been inhibited they transmit different messages. This can affect the libido.

Q: I've heard that the sense of smell becomes keener after chemotherapy. Is this true?

A: Yes. After chemotherapy some patients have a keener sense of smell and a greater sensitivity to odors.

Q: Why do you lose your appetite during chemotherapy?

A: Appetite is an interesting phenomenon. The chemotherapy, by design, kills off rapidly growing cells because they are the ones related to breast cancer. Because the taste cells are fast growing they are destroyed also. It takes a while for the taste buds to mature. Unfortunately, at about day twenty-one when they have fully matured it is usually time for another chemo treatment. So, they are destroyed just as they become completely viable. Hence, the lack of appetite. The longer the chemotherapy regimen, the longer the diminished appetite because nothing tastes good.

Q: I have heard that people have dental problems after cancer. Is this true, and, if so, why?

A: From most of the literature that I have read, dental problems are part and parcel of the cancer experience. Specifically, chemotherapy is the culprit. It is recommended that all dental work, including teeth cleaning, be completed prior to treatment. If it is not possible, as was the case with me, then the best hygiene practices are recommended—brushing regularly with a soft toothbrush and gently flossing. The chemicals used in chemotherapy are hard on the teeth. Any preventative measures that will not cause open lesions in the mouth are helpful.

Because I had always taken good care of my teeth I was not prepared for the shock I received about a year after treatment. My dental bill for fillings, root canal, and crowns was over four thousand dollars! As a youngster I had bad teeth, so as an adult I faithfully kept regular six-month checkups, avoided sweets, and rinsed my mouth after eating, whenever possible. Still, the cancer treatment attacked my teeth.

Q: Does your hair come out all at once after chemotherapy?

A: Hair usually comes out in two major phases, beginning at about three weeks after treatment. First about a half to three-quarters of your hair falls out, then in about another week's time the remaining hair falls out. There are exceptions to this, though. For some people, it comes out all at once.

Q: Are you familiar with anyone who has had children since having cancer?

A: As a matter of fact, I am. I have seen young women in their twenties who, after receiving aggressive treatment, were able to have children several years after recovery.

Q: When visiting a breast cancer patient in the hospital, how can I make my visit enjoyable for her?

A: Oftentimes I hear patients say that they feel like their loved ones are just hovering over them, waiting for their death. One thing that I noticed when I started visiting patients was how uncomfortable they were if visitors stood above them, looking into their faces—as if examining a disaster. I try to sit a distance away from patients, where they can see me but I do not appear too large or too threatening. What I suggest to families is that they take along a newspaper, or a book, or something of interest to the patient when they visit. If the patient is undergoing treatment her vision may be sort of blurry, or she may just be too tired to read. Having someone read to her can be very comforting. If a newspaper article looks like it would be of interest, ask her if she would like to hear about it. In my experience, she usually will. Sometimes listening to music with the patient can be relaxing and enjoyable. Most do not want to constantly discuss their illness or aches and pains. They usually appreciate hearing about current events, both in the world at large and in their social circle. Remember, mealtime visits are usually very helpful, as it can ease difficulty with eating. A little diversion is a wonderful thing.

Q: When you had discomfort in your arm, what did you do about putting on a brassiere?

A: When my arm was frozen, I resorted to finding a brassiere that hooked or closed in the front. If you cannot find a suitable front-closing brassiere, have a seamstress alter one for you. It works very well, so well that some women wonder why they did not consider it prior to having a mastectomy. It's so much easier to open and close. When looking for a new bra make sure that it is sturdy enough to support the prostheses or breast form that you use.

Q: What are the best breast prostheses?

A: I recommend the Amoena brand because they have a variety of forms, weights, sizes, and shapes. There are many other companies that provide for the needs of women who have had a mastectomy. You should feel free to look around and check to see what is affordable, feels comfortable, and looks good. Insurance often covers part of the cost of a prosthesis.

Q: What do you think about prophylactic mastectomies?

A: That is a very individual choice. It requires a lot of discussion between a woman and her physician and loved ones. There is less and less data that indicates that if you have cancer in one breast, you will get it in the other. Surgeons are not removing both breasts as much as they used to because there is so much tactile sensitivity in the nipple and breast tissue. Women surgeons, especially, seem to be concerned with saving the breast. The practice of removing both healthy breasts for women at high risk for cancer is considered a radical yet effective preventative option by some researchers.

Q: Should I insist that my children participate in my treatment regimen?

A: In my experience, the families who have coped most successfully have been open and honest with their children, without burdening them with responsibilities that they are ill-equipped to handle. A lot of this depends upon the age of the patient and the children. If the children are young, just informing them of what is going on and offering to let them participate in a part of the treatment is sometimes helpful. It is especially so if the mother has to go out of town and stay at an extended treatment facility while the oncologist monitors her. When the patient is on the twenty-one-day chemotherapy regimen, she may need to stay in the hospital the first three or four days to be sure everything goes well. Sometimes children accompany her. They then get to vicariously share in the experience and also see that their mother is being carefully treated. There are other events that occur in the course of treatment in which children and family can participate.

One of these is when the patient's hair begins to fall out. This is usually traumatic for the whole family. Some children do not even want their mother to remove her wig at home. Often, adults set the emotional tone for the family; if the adults are embarrassed, the children tend to be so also. If the parents are relaxed and have good coping skills, it can be easier for the children.

When I visited friends during the summertime, I would take off my hat or wig. One of my friend's children commented, "Gee, Alice is like Dad. She wears lots of hats." His mother laughed and said, "It's true." I was very pleased and was again reminded that children are very perceptive. Pretending that children do not realize what's going on is a mistake.

Q: What should I do if I think my physician is wrong?

A: With all illnesses, a second opinion is important and you should feel free to ask for it. If you think your physician is wrong, get the opinion of another specialist as soon as possible.

Q: I'm a mental health professional and I would like to develop stronger relationships with physicians. How can I do that?

A: Over the last twenty-five years I have taken a very direct approach in cultivating these alliances. I have contacted physicians to suggest ways in which I could be helpful in the treatment of his or her patients. Often physicians are interested and willing to listen. All physicians want their patients to get better. If a mental health professional can help a patient adjust and prosper, then the physician will gladly refer patients to him or her. I will never forget the high praise I once received from the chief of surgery at a local hospital. He concluded a presentation with: "One of the best things that ever happened to me was Dr. Chang. After I met her and began sending patients her way, I received 80 percent fewer phone calls. She was able to handle situations that perplexed me a great deal. So I am very thankful to her." This is indicative of the kind of relationship that we as psychologists want to develop with physicians.

Q: Should mental health professionals communicate with other caregivers, besides physicians?

A: Yes. Medical people work as a team so it is important that the nurses, aides, and other consulting physicians understand what we are doing. They need to be aware of the results of our work and our contribution to patient care.

Q: When is it okay to cry?

A: It is okay to cry anytime. Tears come at the most unexpected times for the patient as well as for the patient's family and close friends. The source of these tears may be sadness, anger, fear, or joy. Crying is important and being able to cry with someone who is nonjudgmental and supportive can be very healing.

Q: When should a person begin psychotherapy?

A: You should begin psychotherapy whenever you believe it would be helpful. Psychologists are well trained in helping people communicate with others, making suggestions for working with children, and relieving relationship stress. One of the areas in which psychologists are most helpful is in coping with changing family roles.

Most health care providers, especially mental health professionals, know that breast cancer happens to the entire family. They can help you swiftly identify concerns and make adjustments to effectively function within the family. For this, consulting a mental health professional earlier rather than later is a good idea. Sometimes within the family there are too many sensitive feelings and an outside opinion from a caring professional is just what is needed.

In my opinion, we all need psychotherapy sometime in our lives. If your children need to talk with someone, find a professional trained in treating children. Remember that youngsters do not usually possess the vocabulary to express all of their emotions and concerns, so child therapy often uses a variety of action and play techniques for helping children to communicate.

Q: *How is self-esteem affected by breast cancer?*

A: Individual differences abound, but in general the longer the illness, the greater the impact on self-esteem. Often, patients feel inadequate and insecure because of their illness. But there is hope. With the help of a competent professional you can learn the coping techniques that will help you feel better about yourself and your life.

Q: What about support systems for breast cancer patients? What are your suggestions?

A: Generally speaking, joining a support group of breast cancer patients during and after treatment is very helpful. Support groups for more specific populations can also be a good resource. They are designed to deal with the particular needs of their members.

Q: What are some of the more common issues with long-term recovery?

A: First and foremost is the issue of recurrence—will it happen, when will it happen, and what will I do if it happens? Another issue is the change in body image. Feelings about body image are very individual. Some people don't care so much because they feel that losing their breast(s) is an easy trade off when the alternative may be premature death or susceptibility to recurrence. For others the change in their body becomes a major issue. Most of the time I am okay with only having one breast. Feelings of loss and grief are common in long-term recovery. We have suddenly become painfully aware of our mortality. I have had clients who become overly sensitive to the problems of those around them. They were unable to discern which problems were worthy of their energy and which were not, and often neglected their own needs. Establishing healthy boundaries is crucial. In my opinion, one area that has not received the attention it deserves is changes in sexuality. This is a very important part of a person's life and perhaps because I am single, I neglect to talk about it enough. There are many professionals that deal specifically with this issue. There are many skilled in dealing with our changes in sexuality and our feelings because of this. A psychologist or primary care-giver should be able to provide referrals, and the APA has a help line that can also provide them: 800-964-2000.

Q: What happens when there is a recurrence?

A: The first thing is to remember that we all live in fear of aches, pains, and different body sensations, which we remember from the first time we had cancer. Patients need to attend to these feelings, but not overreact to them. Consult a physician whenever you have a concern about any physical change. Sometimes doctors are so busy that patients must insist that they get the attention they deserve. If indeed there is a recurrence, then it is time to make some decisions about which course of action to take. It is not unusual for patients who have recurrences to consider not getting treated again. Depending on how thorough treatment was the first time, or if they had a bone marrow transplant, they may really be skittish about any further treatment. Talking about life, what you expect of it, one's age, and support system is really important in making this decision. It needs to be made by the patient and patient's family, with the advice of a doctor. Ask your doctor how much time you have to think about it.

Q: Is breast cancer really debilitating?

A: The amount of disability varies according to the individual. In many cases it is debilitating and in many cases it is not. It depends upon when the disease was discovered, the type of the disease, the type of treatment administered, and the stage of the disease. So a diagnosis of breast cancer does not fall neatly into one category. However, it is a chronic illness and one lives with the fear of recurrence from the day of the first diagnosis. Many women live with a generalized fear from listening to stories in the news media. But this is not a reason to stop living. On the contrary, it is a reason to go forward and value each day as it comes.

Q: Why do you consider cancer a chronic illness?

A: I use a broad definition of chronic illness: those that are prolonged and do not resolve spontaneously and are rarely completely cured. For me, the defining criteria for chronic illness is the unknown. With breast cancer it is unknown when and if the cancer will reoccur, and where in the body it will appear. It becomes a chronic problem because it is a fear that most of us live with for the rest of our lives. For many of us, every pain becomes a symptom of recurrence. In some cases the emotional reaction is much greater than the physical one. Sometimes the well-intentioned advice given in self-help books leads people to obsessively monitor and worry about the effects of their emotions. I cannot over-emphasize that the effects of chronic illness differ in degree from person to person. I recommend a good book published by the APA, entitled *Managing Chronic Illness: A Biopsychosocial Approach*, edited by Nicassio and Smith. It focuses on various diseases of the twentieth century.

Q: Do more divorces occur because of breast cancer?

A: In days gone by it was believed that breast cancer caused divorce. In reality, there were usually marital difficulties prior to the wife developing breast cancer. In my experience most couples become closer, more supportive of each other, and learn to look at the more positive aspects of their relationship. They usually make some kind of commitment to work out unresolved issues. This does not mean that they no longer get angry and frustrated with each other. One of the things that family members, and especially husbands, complain about is that the breast cancer patient has become more demanding, more assertive, and, in general, more difficult. In fact, this is probably true. The breast cancer survivor often becomes more willing to advocate for herself. Hallelujah! The contrast in behavior might seem pronounced if she has not spoken out in the past. Because there is a lot of resentment, words and expressions can come out in an awkward manner and sometimes can seem angry or malicious when they are not intended in that manner. Sometimes, though, the anger is quite intentional. This often leads to finding a place for its expression within the bounds of the relationship. The same dynamic applies to couples dealing with breast cancer as for their cancer-free counterparts. If both parties want to make the relationship work, they will make it work. If there are other reasons why it won't work then they will continue to be there until they are resolved.

Q: What do you know about breast cancer in males?

A: According to the National Cancer Institute, male breast cancer is pretty rare, with less than 1 percent of all breast cancers occurring in men. Because it is so uncommon, it has been difficult for researchers to accumulate extensive data. Men are generally somewhat older than women at the time of diagnosis and the disease is more often in an advanced stage. A painless lump is usually discovered by the man, and that is the most common first symptom, although not the only one. Men are more likely to have nipple discharge (especially bloody discharge), nipple retraction, and ulcerated skin. The lump typically appears beneath the areola, where breast tissue is concentrated. About half of the men with breast cancer have palpable axillary lymph nodes. The fact that male breast cancer often spreads locally before diagnosis may be due to the smallness of the breast so that cancer can more easily invade the skin and chest wall. Also, since many tumors are centered around the areola, this may provide the disease with easy access to the internal mammary glands and lymph pathways.

The diagnosis is typically made between the ages of sixty and seventy, although men can be affected at any age. Diagnostic procedures are similar to those used for women and include medical history, physical exam, mammography, and thermography. A definitive diagnosis is made with biopsy and the prognosis depends upon the stage and extent of the disease at diagnosis. Men are commonly treated with surgery for primary disease and usually receive hormone therapy for advanced cases. More men than women respond to hormone therapy. Men are also less likely to develop cancer later in the other breast, but more likely to have had or get a second kind of cancer.

Men and their physicians do not regularly examine their breasts, and when male patients discover signs of cancer they tend to wait before seeing a physician. Some men may feel embarrassed about the possibility of having breast cancer and be reluctant to admit its presence.

Q: Are you familiar with workplace discrimination against breast cancer patients?

A: Nowadays a lot of breast cancer patients continue to work at least part-time, even as they undergo treatment. One common difficulty is that the employer and colleagues do not realize that the employee is sick because she continues to look fairly normal. Often patients do their best to keep up appearances. This results in those around them not appreciating how much they are struggling. The employee is also expected to do well and continue to carry the same load she did before diagnosis. Employer insensitivity can lead to workplace discrimination. Employers may not acknowledge that recovering patients need special consideration because they are tired or in pain.

Q: Do you recommend genetic testing?

A: Genetic testing is a complicated issue. There is only a very small percentage of breast cancer patients that carry the gene. The legal, ethical, and social implications of genetic testing have not yet been carefully explored. These include the possibilities of job discrimination, insurability of the patient or the patient's family, and how well the family will deal with it. There are lots of issues that need to be thoroughly examined in detail before some effective protocol can be developed.

Q: What financial impact has cancer had on you and your clients?

A: This is a complex question. Personally, I was not working and was in transition, having just moved to a new location when I was diagnosed. I was fortunate because I had APA income protection insurance for disability. When I received my diagnosis, I soon became eligible to receive benefits. In addition, because I had paid into Social Security regularly and my diagnosis was severe, I received Social Security disability after six months (the amount of the benefit is dependent on how much you have contributed to the system). I was initially able to pay my living expenses but not my medical and dental bills Fortunately, when I finally was able to get back on my feet and start all over again, I was able to refinance my house, take out a business and professional loan, and make payments against any outstanding balances.

One of the things that happens during cancer is that people expect the patient to be able to maintain the same lifestyle that she had in the past. For many people, including myself, this was just impossible. I was often reminded of my poor starving-student days.

Q: If you do not have money, what do you do for fun or distractions?

A: Good question. I remember when I went to the Behavioral Health Conference and listened to cancer survivors talk about what they had done just before their bone marrow transplants, or as a celebration of life after treatment. They did things such as scuba diving and traveling to Alaska. It all sounded very expensive to me. Yes, I would like to do those things too, but they were not within my budget.

However, good things do happen if we are open to them. A very dear colleague of mine asked me while I was sick, "If you could do anything you wished when you get better, what would it be?" All I could think of was that the Super Bowl was going to be in Phoenix next January and my favorite teams were probably going to play in it—the Kansas City Chiefs and the San Francisco Forty-Niners. He replied, "That's interesting." Super Bowl XXX came to Phoenix and I got a phone call, "Alice, they're not your teams, but do you still want to go to the Super Bowl?" I was so excited! It was the Dallas Cowboys and Pittsburgh Steelers, but I still had a great time. I took my hairdresser, Rudi, who is a diehard Cowboys fan. I was still really weak from chemotherapy but we went just the same. It was nice to do a favor for Rudi since she had helped to make me presentable many times.

Some fun things don't cost money, but take more time and effort to appreciate. There are many small things in life to anticipate and enjoy: sitting down to a meal without feeling nauseated, or when we can honestly reply, "Great," to the question, "How do you feel?" The cards, the flowers, the phone messages, the freedom to make ones' own decisions again—these are all uplifting. Also, for some of us, short trips are fun. Doing something for enjoyment that does not stress the finances too much is more prudent, especially when you do not know what the future holds. Single women have to be shrewd with their money because they have no one to ease the financial burden.

Simple pleasures have taken on a priceless significance to me. On a cloudy day watching the sunset with my neighbors I was reminded of life's beauty and that the earth continues to rotate—the sun continues to rise in the east and set in the west. Each sunset reminds me that I have lived for one more day.

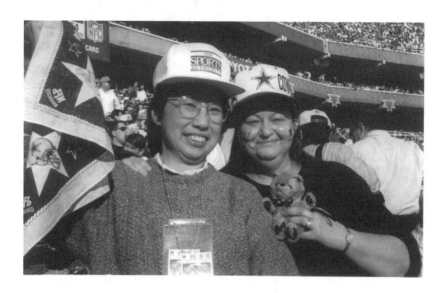

Me and Rudi at the Super Bowl

Resources

The world of information services for the breast cancer patient is indeed a rich and expansive smorgasbord. If you have a home or office computer, the Internet offers endless avenues of discovery regarding the latest research, listservs, chat rooms, shopping, electronic mail, and physician and hospital directories. From these resources I readily found personal stories, references to creative works, and reading materials. The threat of isolation is diminishing as breast cancer patients from around the globe can compare notes and experiences while offering one another emotional support. Real friendships often grow out of these virtual encounters. Even if you are limited to telephone, standard mail service, local libraries, bookstores, and clinics, many helpful services exist.

In this day and age, computers seem to loom large. However, if you are like me, you are in the infancy of your online life. I have discovered that those not familiar with or comfortable using a computer can get helpful hints and guidance from a variety of resources like the local library, community college, or senior center. Avail yourself of all your resources.

In this section, I have listed some references that I believe will be useful, whether you are a patient, family member, or professional caregiver.

Agencies and Organizations

Academy for Cancer Wellness. 6616 E. Carondelet Dr., Tucson, AZ 85710. Phone: (520) 722-4581; fax: 520-722-4582. Among other services, publishes a newsletter entitled, *Cancer Wellness News.*

American Cancer Society, Inc. 1599 Clifton Rd. NE, Atlanta, GA 30329. Phone: (800) 227-2345 or (404) 320-3333; Web site: http://www.cancer.org.

American Institute for Cancer Research. 1759 R St. NW, Washington, DC 20009. Phone: (800) 843-8114 or (202) 328-7744; fax: (202) 328-7226; e-mail: admin@aud.org.

American Psychological Association. 750 First Street, NE, Washington, DC 20002. Phone: (202) 336-5500 or (800) 374-2721 (U.S. and Canada); fax: (202) 336-5568; Web site http://www.apa.org/.

The Bosom Buddy Club. Joan Dawson, 1057 Columbia Pl., Boulder, CO 80303. Phone: (303) 494-8252. For women who are considering prophylactic mastectomy.

Cancer Care Center of Southern Arizona. 2625 N. Craycroft Rd, #200, Tucson AZ 85718. Phone: (520) 324-2409; fax: (520) 324-2454; Web site: http://www.usoncology.com.

The Cancer Hotline. 4435 Main St., Kansas City, MO 64111. Phone: (800) 433-0464 or (816) 932-8453; fax: (816) 931-7486; e-mail: hotline@hrblock.com.

Cerelle Center for Mammography. 3100 N Campbell Ave., #103, Tucson, AZ 85719 Phone: (520) 325-3000.

Corporate Angel Network, Inc. (CAN). One Loop Rd., Westchester County Airport, White Plains, NY 10604. Phone (914) 328-1313. They provide free air transportation for cancer patients traveling to or from recognized treatment centers in the U.S. without regard to their financial resources.

Health Sciences Education Center. Carter Hall Lakes, Millwood, VA 22646. Phone: (540) 837-2100; fax (540) 837-1813.

Kids Konnected. P.O. Box 603, Trabuco Canyon, CA 92687. Phone: (800) 899-2866, within CA; (714) 381-4334, outside of CA; fax: (949) 582-3989; Web site: http://www.kidskonnected.org;

e-mail: JWH@kidskonnected.org. They provide friendship, education, and support to kids who have a parent with cancer.

Mammacare. P.O. Box 15748, Gainesville, FL 32604. Phone: (800) 626-2273; e-mail: mammatech@mail.com. MammaCare offers a Personal Learning System that enables a woman to learn a research-based breast self-exam method in the convenience of her own home. Professional training programs are also available.

Mautner Project for Lesbians with Cancer. 1707 L Street NW, Suite 500, Washington, DC 20036. Phone: (202) 332-5536; fax: (202) 332-0662; e-mail: mautner@mautnerproject.org.

The National Alliance of Breast Cancer Organizations (NABCO). 9 E. 37th St., 10th Floor, New York, NY 10016. Phone: (888) 80-NABCO or (212) 719-0154; fax: (212) 689-1213; Web site: http://www.nabco.org/; e-mail: nabcoinfo@aol.com.

National Breast Cancer Coalition. 1707 L St. NW, Suite 1060, Washington, DC 20036. Phone: (202) 296-7477; fax: (202) 265-6854; Web site: http://www.natlbcc.org; e-mail: info@natlbcc.org.

National Cancer Institute. 9000 Rockville Pike, Bldg. 31, Rm. 10A16, Bethesda, MD 20892-0001. Phone: (800) 4-CANCER or (301) 496-4000; Web site: http://www.nci.nih.gov.

National Coalition for Cancer Survivorship (NCSS). 1010 Wayne Ave., 5th Floor, Silver Spring, MD 20910. Phone: (888) 937-6227; fax: (301) 365-9670; e-mail: info@cansearch.org.

National High Risk Registry. Strang-Cornell Breast Center, 428 E. 72nd St., New York, NY 10021. Phone: (212) 794-4900. They are dedicated to research to prevent cancer and promote cure through early detection.

National Lymphedema Network. 2211 Post St., Suite 404, San Francisco, CA 94115-3427. Phone: (800) 541-3259 or (415) 921-1306; fax: (415) 921-4284; e-mail: nln@lymphnet.org.

National Patient Air Transport Helpline (NPATH). P.O. Box 1960, Manassas, VA 20108-0804. Phone: (800) 296-1217, within the U.S.; (757)318-9145, outside of the U.S.; fax: (757) 318-9107; Web site: http://www.npath.org; e-mail: npath@aol.com. They make referrals to charitable and discounted patient medical air transport.

National Self-Help Clearinghouse. City University of New York, 25 W. 43rd St., Rm. 620, New York, NY 10036. Phone: (212) 354-8525.

National Society of Genetic Counselors, Inc. 233 Canterbury Dr., Wallingford, PA 19086-6617. Phone: (610) 879-7608; e-mail: nsgc@aol.com.

S.D. Pain Management Clinic. 3703 Camino del Rio S., Suite 210, San Diego, CA 92108. Phone: (619) 640-5555; fax (619) 640-5550; e-mail djs@sadiegopain.com.

Vital Options Telesupport Cancer Network. The Group Room Radio Talk Show, P.O. Box 19233, Encino, CA 91416-9233. Phone: (818) 788-5225; fax: (818) 788-5260. Founded and hosted by a breast cancer survivor, this weekly syndicated call-in cancer talk show links callers with other patients, long-term survivors, family members, physicians, researchers, and therapists.

Y-Me National Breast Cancer Organization. 212 W. Van Buren St., Chicago, IL 60607. Phone: Twenty-four hour hotline (800) 221-2141 or (312) 986-8228; twenty-four hour Spanish (800) 986-9505; fax: (312) 294-8597; e-mail: help@y-me.org.

YWCA of the U.S.A. Office of Women's Health Initiative, ENCOREplus Program, 624 9th St. NW, 3rd Floor, Washington DC 20001-5303. Phone: (800) 953-7587 or (202) 628-3636; fax: (202) 783-7123; e-mail: cgould@ywca.org. This program is designed to meet the needs of medically underserved women for early detection, education, breast and cervical screening, and support services.

Reading Material

Album, Mitch. 1997. *Tuesdays with Morrie*. New York: Doubleday.

American Cancer Society. 1997. *Breast Health Guide*. Florida Division of the ACS.

American Cancer Society & National Cancer Institute. 1992. *Questions and Answers About Pain Control: A Guide for People with Cancer and Their Families.*

American Psychological Association. 1993. *Breast Cancer: A Psychological Treatment Manual.* Phoenix, AZ.

Beck, Aaron T. 1988. *Love Is Never Enough: How Couples Can Overcome Misunderstandings, Resolve Conflicts, and Solve Relationship Problems Through Cognitive Therapy.* New York: Harper & Row Publishers.

Benson, Herbert, with Marg Stark. 1996. *Timeless Healing.* New York: Scribner.

Bourne, Edmund J. 1990. *The Anxiety and Phobia Workbook. A Step-by-Step Program For Curing Yourself of Extreme Anxiety, Panic Attacks, and Phobias.* Oakland, CA: New Harbinger Publications.

Butler, Gillian, and Tony Hope. 1995. *Managing Your Mind.* New York: Oxford University Press.

Cantor, Dorothy, Toni Bernay and Jean Stoess. 1992. *Women in Power: The Secrets of Leadership.* New York: Houghton-Mifflin.

Caudill, Margaret A. 1995. *Managing Pain Before it Manages You.* New York: The Guilford Press.

Coping with Cancer magazine. P. O. Box 682268, Franklin, TN 37068-2268. Phone 615-790-2400; fax 615-794-0179; e-mail: Copingmag@aol.com.

Cousins, Norman. 1989. *Head First: The Biology of Hope.* New York: E. P. Dutton.

Davis, Martha, Elizabeth Robbins Eshelman, and Mathew McKay. 1995. *The Relaxation and Stress Reduction Workbook.* Fourth Edition. Oakland, CA: New Harbinger Publications.

Deardorff, William W. and John L. Reeves II. 1997. *Preparing for Surgery: A Mind-Body Approach to Enhance Healing and Recovery.* Oakland, CA: New Harbinger Publications.

Dreher, Henry. 1995. *The Immune Power Personality. 7 Traits You Can Develop to Stay Healthy.* New York: Dutton.

Dorfman, Elena. 1994. *The C-Word: Teenagers and Their Families Living with Cancer.* Portland, OR NewSage Press.

Epping-Jordan, JoAnne E., et. al. 1999. Psychological adjustment in breast cancer: processes of emotional distress. *Health Psychology* 18:315–326.

Field, Tiffany M. 1998. Massage therapy effects. *American Psychologist* 53:1270–1281.

Fletcher, Suzanne W., Michael S. O'Malley, and Leslie A. Bunce. 1985. Physicians' abilities to detect lumps in silicone breast models. *Journal of the American Medical Association* 253:2224–2228.

Fletcher, Suzanne W., Michael S. O'Malley, JoAnne L. Earp, Timothy M. Morgan, Shao Lin, and Darrah Degnan. 1990. How best to teach women breast self-examination: a randomized controlled trial. *Annals of Internal Medicine* 112:772–779.

Fulford, Robert C., with Gene Stone. 1997. *Dr. Fulford's Touch of Life: The Healing Power of the Natural Life Force.* New York: Simon and Schuster.

Gersh, Wayne D., William L. Golden, and David M. Robbins. 1997. *Mind over Malignancy: Living with Cancer.* Oakland, CA: New Harbinger Publications.

Goodwin, Aurelie Jones, and Mark E. Agronin. 1997. *A Woman's Guide to Overcoming Sexual Fear and Pain.* Oakland, CA: New Harbinger Publications.

Haber, Sandra, Catherine Acuff, and Lauren Ayers. 1995. *Breast Cancer: A Psychological Treatment Manual.* Springer Pub. Co.

Hoffman, C., D. Rice, D. and H-Y Sun. 1996. Persons with chronic conditions:Their prevalence and cost. *Journal of the American Medical Association* 276:1473–1479.

Kiecolt-Glaser, Janice K., Gayle G. Gage, Phillip T. Marucha, Robert C. MacCallum, and Ronald Glaser. 1998. Psychological influences on surgical recovery: perspectives from psychoneuroimmunology. *American Psychologist* 53:1209–1218.

Klauser, Henriette Anne. 1995. *Putting Your Heart on Paper: Staying Connected in a Loose-Ends World.* New York: Bantam Books.

Lee, Evelyn. 1997. *Working with Asian Americans, A Guide for Clinicians.* New York: The Guilford Press.

Lorig, Kate, Dr. P.H., Holman, Halsted, M.D., Sobel, David, M.D., Laurent, Diana, M.P.H., Gonzalez, Virginia, M.P.H., and Marian Minor, R.P.T., Ph.D. 1994. *Living a Healthy Life with Chronic Conditions.* Palo, Alto, CA: Bull Publishing Co.

Love, Susan M., with Karen Lindsey. 1990. *Dr. Susan Love's Breast Book.* New York: Random House.

————. 1997 *Dr. Susan Love's Hormone Book: Making Informed Choices about Menopause.* New York: Random House.

McDaniel, Susan H., and Thomas Campbell, eds. 1999. Families, system & health (special edition). *Journal of Collaborative Family Healthcare.* 17:1.

McGrath, Ellen. 1992. *When Feeling Bad Is Good.* New York: Henry Holt and Company.

McKay, Judith, and Nancee Hirano. 1998. *The Chemotherapy and Radiation Therapy Survival Guide.* Oakland, CA: New Harbinger Publications.

McKay, Matthew, Martha Davis, and Patrick Fanning. 1995. *Messages: The Communication Skills Book.* Oakland, CA: New Harbinger Publications.

McKay, Matthew, Patrick Fanning, and Kim Paleg. 1994. *Couple Skills: Making Your Relationship Work.* Oakland, CA: New Harbinger Publications.

Moyers, Bill. 1993. *Healing and the Mind.* New York: Main Street Books, Doubleday.

Murray, Bridget. 1998. Vertical-strips method for breast self-exam uses 'touch intelligence,' *APA Monitor,* December, 12-13.

Myss, Caroline. 1997. *Why People Don't Heal and How They Can.* NY: Harmony Books.

Myss, Caroline, with C. Norman Shealy. 1998. *The Creation of Health: The Emotional, Psychological, and Spiritual Responses That Promote Health and Healing.* New York: Crown Publishing Group.

National Cancer Institute. 1990. *After Breast Cancer: A Guide to Followup Care.* NIH Publication.

National Cancer Institute. 1992. *Eating Hints: Recipes and Tips for Better Nutrition during Cancer Treatment.* NIH Publication No. 92-2079.

National Cancer Institute. 1993. *Understanding Breast Changes: A Health Guide for All Women.* NCI Publications.

National Cancer Institute. 1995. *Understanding Gene Testing.* NIH Publication. December.

National Institutes of Health—National Cancer Institute. 1993. *Chemotherapy and You: A Guide to Self-help during Treatment.* NIH Publication No. 97-1136.

National Institutes of Health. 1994. *Management of Cancer Pain, Clinical Practice Guideline,* number 9. March.

National Institutes of Health—National Cancer Institute. 1992. *Radiation Therapy and You: A Guide to Self-Help During Treatment.* NIH Publication No. 92-2227.

Newsweek. 1999. Health for life. Special Edition. Newsweek Inc., 251 West 57th Street, New York, NY. Spring/Summer.

Nicassio, P. M., and T. W. Smith, eds. 1995. *Managing Chronic Illness: A Biopsychosocial Approach.* Washington, DC: American Psychological Association.

Northrup, Christiane. 1994. *Women's Bodies, Women's Wisdom: Creating Physical and Emotional Health and Healing.* New York: Bantam Books.

Ornish, Dean. 1997. *Love & Survival.* New York: HarperCollins.

Pennebaker, James W. 1997. *Opening Up: The Healing Power of Expressing Emotions.* New York: The Guilford Press.

People Weekly. 1998. Surviving breast cancer (speical report). 52-74. Customer Service at 1-800-541-9000. October 26.

Pearsall, Paul. 1987. *Superimmunity. Master Your Emotions & Improve Your Health.* New York: McGraw-Hill.

Rico, Garbriele Lusser. 1991. *Pain and Possibility: Writing Your Way Through Personal Crisis.* New York: JP Tarcher.

Roberts, M. Susan, and Gerard J. Jansen. 1997. *Living with ADD: A Workbook for Adults.* Oakland, CA: New Harbinger Publications.

Saunders, Kathryn J., Carol A. Pilgrim, and Henry S. Pennypacker. 1986. Increased proficiency of search in breast self-examination. *Cancer* 58:2531–2537.

Schwartz, Marc D., et al. July 1999. Distress, personality, and mammography utilization among women with a family history of breast cancer. *Health Psychology* 18: 327–345.

Segal, Jeanne. 1997. *Raising Your Emotional Intelligence*. New York: Henry Holt.

Seligman, E.P. Martin. 1991. *Learned Optimism*. New York: Alfred A. Knopf.

Seligman, E.P. Martin. 1994. *What You Can Change & What You Can't*. New York: Alfred A. Knopf.

Seligman, E.P. Martin, with Karen Reivich, Lisa Jaycox, and Jane Gillham. 1995. *The Optimistic Child*. New York: Houghton-Mifflin.

Siegel, Bernie S. 1990. *Love, Medicine and Miracles: Lessons Learned About Self-Healing from a Surgeon's Experience with Exceptional Patients*. New York: Harper Perennial Library.

Somkin, Carol P. 1993. Improving the effectiveness of breast self-examination in the early detection of breast cancer: A selective review of the literature. *Nurse Practitioner Forum* 4:76–84.

Spiegel, David. 1993. *Living Beyond Limits*. New York: Times Books.

Tomlinson, Theresa. 1997. *Dancing through the Shadows*. Orlando, FL: DK Publishing Incorp.

Touchette, N. Holtzman, Neal A. Davis, Jessica G. Feetham Suzzane. 1997. *Toward the 21st Century: Incorporating Genetics into Primary Health Care*. New York: Cold Spring Harbor Laboratory Press.

U.S. Department of Health and Human Services. 1994. *Management of Cancer Pain: Clinical Practice Guideline*. AHCPR Publication. March.

Valley, Mary Jo, J. Ellen Doice, and Madeline Canzani. 1996. *Please Don't Go*. Unionville, NY: Royal Fireworks Printing Company.

Weil, Andrew. 1995. *Spontaneous Healing: How to Discover and Enhance Your Body's Natural Ability to Maintain and Heal Itself*. New York: Alfred A. Knopf.

Wittig, Susan Albert. 1996. *Writing from Life: Telling Your Soul's Story*. New York: Tarcher/Putnam.

Internet Resources

http://www.aath.org/. American Association for Therapeutic Humor. An organization committed to advancing our knowledge and understanding of humor and laughter as they relate to healing and well-being.

http://www.ac.org/. The Alpha Center. Established in 1976, this is a non-profit and non-partisan health policy center that helps public and private sector clients respond to health care challenges.

http://www.acor.org/. The Association of Cancer Online Resources, Inc. (ACOR). This is a non-profit patient advocacy organization founded in 1996 by Gilles Frydman after his wife was diagnosed with breast cancer. ACOR's mission is to develop, support, and represent Internet-based resources providing high quality, up-to-date information and support to cancer patients, their loved ones and caretakers, regardless of geographical location or type of cancer, and to provide open communication channels between and among patients, health professionals, and research scientists.

http://www.ahsr.org. The Association for Health Services Research (AHSR). A non-profit, tax-exempt organization, the association is governed by a board of directors elected by and responsive to the membership. Its primary mission is to increase the contribution that health services research makes to improve the health care system and health status of Americans.

http://www.amwa-doc.org/. The American Medical Women's Association. This is a national organization of women physicians and medical students. They are dedicated to promoting women's health, improving the professional development and personal well-being of its members, and increasing the influence of women in all aspects of the medical profession.

http://www.avoncrusade.com/. Founded in 1993, this is the largest corporate supporter of breast health programs in America.

http://www.best.com/~mlsp/resource.html. The Mothers' Living Stories Project. They provide information on San Francisco Bay area support groups, and written materials for parents living with cancer.

http://www.blochcancer.org. R. A. Bloch Cancer Foundation, Inc.

http://www.bmtnews.org//newsletters/issue34/helping.html. This article helps adults discuss cancer with children.

http://www.breastcancer.net/cgi/bcn.main.wcgi. BreastCancerNet. Each day BreastCancerNet searches dozens of news services for breast cancer related news and articles, and links are posted to these stories on the site. They also provide free e-mail notification of breaking breast cancer–related news and new article postings.

http://cancernet.nci.nih.gov/. CancerNet. CancerNet was created to provide up-to-date, accurate cancer information from the National Cancer Institute's Office of Cancer Information, Communication, and Education.

http://www.cancer.ucdmc.ucdavis.edu/brstsupp.htm. UC Davis Cancer Center. Breast cancer support groups in the United States and Canada.

http://www.candlelighters.ca/. Candlelighters Childhood Cancer Foundation Canada. This organization has put a large resource catalog online, including categories for when a parent dies, when a parent has cancer, siblings, bereavement, and adolescents.

http://www.celebratinglife.org/. Celebrating Life Foundation. The foundation promotes breast cancer awareness specifically geared toward women of color.

http://cnacerfatigue.org/. This Oncology Nursing Society Website is an interactive, confidential Internet resource where cancer patients and caregivers can ask personal questions about cancer fatigue to oncology nurses.

http://www.consumersunion.org/. Consumer's Union. This site provides informative and educational materials developed by Consumer's Union's advocacy offices on a variety of consumer issues, including health-care, financial services, food safety, product safety, and more.

http://darkwing.uoregon.edu/~jbonine/bc_sources.html   Jon Bonine's extensive compilation. Email: jbonine@oregon.uoregon.edu.

http://healthlink.mcw.edu/article/917588037.html. The Medical College of Wisconsin's Health Link offers this article about communication for couples dealing with breast cancer. It is written by Ross E. Carter, Ph.D., Associate Professor of Psychiatry and Behavioral Medicine, and Charlene A. Carter, Ph.D.

http://www.infomedical.com/idx/337.stm. The Medical Business Search Engine.

http://www.komenorg/. The Susan G. Komen Breast Cancer Foundation. This website contains over a hundred pages of general breast health information, along with specific areas that address the needs of special audiences, including health cancer survivors and their friends and families, the media, and the medical and scientific communities.

http://ktf.org. Court Jesters page for Humor. Email: ktf@ktf.org.

http://mel.lib.mi.us/. The Michigan Electronic Library offers a quick way to find resources for children.

http://www.nccn.org. National Comprehensive Cancer Network. A coalition of cancer care institutions and health care providers, working to develop and implement oncology practice guidelines and data collection. Also can be reached at: 888-909-NCCN.

http://www.nci.nih.gov. National Cancer Institute (NCI). Also can be reached at (800) 4-CANCER (1-800-422-6237).

http://www.oncolink.upenn.edu. OncoLink. University of Pennsylvania Cancer Center, 3400 Spruce Street, 2 Donner, Philadelphia, PA 19104. Phone: (215) 349-8895; fax: (215) 349-5445; e-mail: editors@oncolink.upenn.edu. Oncolink was founded in 1994 by Penn cancer specialists with a mission to help cancer patients, families, health care professionals, and the general public get accurate cancer-related information at no charge.

Patient Products

Alice Rae's Intimate Apparel. 6212 E. Speedway Tucson, AZ 85712. Phone: (520) 745-5878.

Betty Schwartz's Intimate Boutique. Phone: (847) 432-0220; fax: (847) 432-9415; e-mail: info@bettyschwartzs.com/. A fine specialty store for women's intimate apparel and a resource for name-brand lingerie and post-surgical fittings, featuring Amoena breast forms and bras. Three Chicago-area locations.

Land's End Mastectomy Swimwear. Phone: (800) 388-3677; e-mail: www.landsend.com.

Mary's Place Boutique. 4826 Shallow Creek Dr., Kennesaw, GA 30144. Phone: (770) 517-7291; Web site: http://www. marysplace.com.

Reflections of Symmetry. Web site: http://www.fwp.net/ ReflectionsofSymmetry/reflections/promotio.htm. They offers breast forms, mastectomy bras, wigs, hats, and Amoena swimwear.

The Ungame—Families Version. A non-competitive family communication game with a variety of versions. Contact Talicor, Inc. Phone: (702) 655-4377.

More New Harbinger Titles

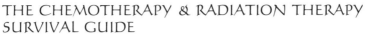

THE CHEMOTHERAPY & RADIATION THERAPY SURVIVAL GUIDE
Lets you know what to expect at each stage of treatment and tells you exactly what you can do to prevent or minimize side-effects.
Item CHEM Paperback $14.95

MIND OVER MALIGNANCY
A step-by-step program shows you how to cope with stress and depression, control pain and side-effects, and improve your quality of life.
Item MALI Paperback, $12.95

PERIMENOPAUSE
This self-care guide helps women cope with symptoms and assure health and vitality in the years ahead.
Item PERI Paperback $16.95

WINNING AGAINST RELAPSE
How to monitor symptoms and respond to them in a way that reduces or eliminates the possibility of relapse.
Item WIN Paperback $14.95

TAKING CONTROL OF TMJ
Learn how to improve jaw functioning, relieve pain, eliminate harmful habits, and improve diet and exercise habits.
Item TMJ Paperback, $13.95

FIBROMYALGIA & CHRONIC MYOFASCIAL PAIN SYNDROME
This comprehensive patient guide teaches you how to identify trigger points, cope with chronic pain and sleep problems, and deal with the numbing effects of "fibrofog."
Item FMS Paperback, $19.95

Call **toll-free 1-800-748-6273** to order. Have your Visa or Mastercard number ready. Or send a check for the titles you want to New Harbinger Publications, 5674 Shattuck Avenue, Oakland, CA 94609. Include $3.80 for the first book and 75¢ for each additional book to cover shipping and handling. (California residents please include appropriate sales tax.) Allow four to six weeks for delivery.

Prices subject to change without notice.

Some Other New Harbinger Self-Help Titles

Virtual Addiction, $12.95
After the Breakup, $13.95
Why Can't I Be the Parent I Want to Be?, $12.95
The Secret Message of Shame, $13.95
The OCD Workbook, $18.95
Tapping Your Inner Strength, $13.95
Binge No More, $14.95
When to Forgive, $12.95
Practical Dreaming, $12.95
Healthy Baby, Toxic World, $15.95
Making Hope Happen, $14.95
I'll Take Care of You, $12.95
Survivor Guilt, $14.95
Children Changed by Trauma, $13.95
Understanding Your Child's Sexual Behavior, $12.95
The Self-Esteem Companion, $10.95
The Gay and Lesbian Self-Esteem Book, $13.95
Making the Big Move, $13.95
How to Survive and Thrive in an Empty Nest, $13.95
Living Well with a Hidden Disability, $15.95
Overcoming Repetitive Motion Injuries the Rossiter Way, $15.95
What to Tell the Kids About Your Divorce, $13.95
The Divorce Book, Second Edition, $15.95
Claiming Your Creative Self: True Stories from the Everyday Lives of Women, $15.95
Six Keys to Creating the Life You Desire, $19.95
Taking Control of TMJ, $13.95
What You Need to Know About Alzheimer's, $15.95
Winning Against Relapse: A Workbook of Action Plans for Recurring Health and Emotional Problems, $14.95
Facing 30: Women Talk About Constructing a Real Life and Other Scary Rites of Passage, $12.95
The Worry Control Workbook, $15.95
Wanting What You Have: A Self-Discovery Workbook, $18.95
When Perfect Isn't Good Enough: Strategies for Coping with Perfectionism, $13.95
Earning Your Own Respect: A Handbook of Personal Responsibility, $12.95
High on Stress: A Woman's Guide to Optimizing the Stress in Her Life, $13.95
Infidelity: A Survival Guide, $13.95
Stop Walking on Eggshells, $14.95
Consumer's Guide to Psychiatric Drugs, $16.95
The Fibromyalgia Advocate: Getting the Support You Need to Cope with Fibromyalgia and Myofascial Pain, $18.95
Healing Fear: New Approaches to Overcoming Anxiety, $16.95
Working Anger: Preventing and Resolving Conflict on the Job, $12.95
Sex Smart: How Your Childhood Shaped Your Sexual Life and What to Do About It, $14.95
You Can Free Yourself From Alcohol & Drugs, $13.95
Amongst Ourselves: A Self-Help Guide to Living with Dissociative Identity Disorder, $14.95
Healthy Living with Diabetes, $13.95
Dr. Carl Robinson's Basic Baby Care, $10.95
Better Boundries: Owning and Treasuring Your Life, $13.95
Goodbye Good Girl, $12.95
Fibromyalgia & Chronic Myofascial Pain Syndrome, $19.95
The Depression Workbook: Living With Depression and Manic Depression, $17.95
Self-Esteem, Second Edition, $13.95
Angry All the Time: An Emergency Guide to Anger Control, $12.95
When Anger Hurts, $13.95
Perimenopause, $16.95
The Relaxation & Stress Reduction Workbook, Fourth Edition, $17.95
The Anxiety & Phobia Workbook, Second Edition, $18.95
I Can't Get Over It, A Handbook for Trauma Survivors, Second Edition, $16.95
Messages: The Communication Skills Workbook, Second Edition, $15.95
Thoughts & Feelings, Second Edition, $18.95
Depression: How It Happens, How It's Healed, $14.95
The Deadly Diet, Second Edition, $14.95
The Power of Two, $15.95
Living Without Depression & Manic Depression: A Workbook for Maintaining Mood Stability, $18.95
Couple Skills: Making Your Relationship Work, $14.95
Hypnosis for Change: A Manual of Proven Techniques, Third Edition, $15.95
Letting Go of Anger: The 10 Most Common Anger Styles and What to Do About Them, $12.95
Infidelity: A Survival Guide, $13.95
When Anger Hurts Your Kids, $12.95
Don't Take It Personally, $12.95
The Addiction Workbook, $17.95

Call **toll free, 1-800-748-6273,** or log on to our online bookstore at **www.newharbinger.com** to order. Have your Visa or Mastercard number ready. Or send a check for the titles you want to New Harbinger Publications, Inc., 5674 Shattuck Ave., Oakland, CA 94609. Include $3.80 for the first book and 75¢ for each additional book, to cover shipping and handling. (California residents please include appropriate sales tax.) Allow two to five weeks for delivery.

Prices subject to change without notice.